INTERACTIONS BETWEEN CHINESE HERBAL MEDICINAL PRODUCTS AND ORTHODOX DRUGS

INTERACTIONS BETWEEN CHINESE HERBAL MEDICINAL PRODUCTS AND ORTHODOX DRUGS

Kelvin Chan
School of Pharmacy and Chemistry
Liverpool John Moores University, UK;
Zayed Complex for Herbal Research and Traditional Medicine
Abu Dhabi, United Arab Emirates

and

Lily Cheung
Chung San School of Acupuncture, London, UK

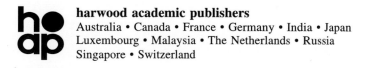

harwood academic publishers
Australia • Canada • France • Germany • India • Japan
Luxembourg • Malaysia • The Netherlands • Russia
Singapore • Switzerland

Amsteldijk 166
1st Floor
1079 LH Amsterdam
The Netherlands

British Library Cataloguing in Publication Data

Chan, Kevin
    Interactions between Chinese herbal medicine products and
    orthodox drugs
    1. Drug interactions 2. Herbs – Therapeutic use – China
    I. Title II. Cheung, Lily
    615.7′045

    ISBN: 90-5702-413-6

CONTENTS

FOREWORD

Chinese herbal medicine is an integral part of traditional Chinese medicine which has a long and distinguished history. The earliest record of Chinese herbal medicine is that prepared by the folklore hero Shen Nong. His 'Herbal Classic of the Divine Plowman' (the *Shen Nong Ben Cao Jing*) which was produced in about 2800 BC, describes the use of over 350 herbal materials. Nearly four thousand years later a monumental work was completed by Li Shi Zhen who compiled a comprehensive pharmacopoeia published in AD 1590. This work entitled '*Ben Cao Gang Mu*' (Compendium of Materia Medica) consisted of 52 volumes and described some 11,000 prescriptions. The general view now is that some 4000 herbs are used from time to time and about 500 are in everyday use (see Chapter 4). The history of the so called orthodox medicines is thus very recent and brief in comparison although the number of orthodox drugs available is very similar.

I remember well visiting the People's Republic of China over ten years ago as an adviser for the World Health Organisation. My brief, together with a fellow adviser from the Region, was to advise on the setting up of a system to monitor the adverse effects of drugs. We were told at an early stage that this should only concern orthodox 'western' drugs, since Chinese traditional medicines, mostly obtained from herbal sources, could not by definition do any harm. Given the long history of benefit from Chinese herbal medicine it is not surprising that such a view should prevail.

Chinese herbal medicine is usually prepared as complex concoctions of plant materials with occasional addition of animal or mineral substances. These are usually boiled together to make a warm concoction which is then consumed orally. The resulting mixture will contain many chemical entities and modern medicinal chemists have been kept busy in trying to identify the ingredient or ingredients through which therapeutic activity is manifested. An example from a field in which I have been slightly involved concerns the traditional medicine Qing Hao, which is prepared from the plant *Artemisia annua L* and which has excellent anti-malarial properties. It is now known the therapeutic activity is vested in a variety of chemical substances such as artemisinine and derivatives such as artemether and artenilic acid. Similar work has identified steroid-like activity in Chinese herbal medicines from which the active substances are being identified.

It is now recognised that Chinese herbal medicines contain potent chemical substances and that these substances have the power to benefit the patients as well as occasionally causing adverse effects depending on the circumstances. It would therefore not be surprising to find that Chinese herbal medicines and orthodox drugs can occasionally interact together to produce both adverse effects and clinical benefit. This book is a comprehensive text aimed at approaching the subject from a modern scientific point of view while concentrating on those areas of clinical relevance. Thus the initial chapters deal with the science behind the dynamics and kinetics of drugs as well as the background to Chinese herbal medicine. While the book identifies a number of interactions it is also recognised that the subject is in its infancy and so the book also addresses the way in which the subject should be studied in the future. It is a fascinating subject that is likely to become of increasing importance in the future. As travel and migration brings a further mixing of the world's cultures, this topic is likely to be of increasing importance to doctors and other health professionals wherever they may be practising. I commend this book to the reader both as an interesting read as well as an important reference text for the future.

Michael Orme
Professor of Pharmacology and Therapeutics
University of Liverpool
UK

PREFACE

This book is written to draw the attention of both the orthodox medicine (OM) and traditional Chinese medicine (TCM) practitioners and other health-care professionals to be cautious about the likelihood of potential benefits, therapeutic failure, or life-threatening adverse effects when Chinese herbal medicine (CHM) products and orthodox drugs or medicinal products are co-administered intentionally or unintentionally. It is common knowledge that patients in some Chinese communities may self-medicate CHM products as food supplements while taking OM drugs. On the other hand, few practitioners may use both OM and CHM products to obtain benefits from the combination of both therapies. This requires expert knowledge of both practices, which have a different basis of diagnosis and treatment methods. At present there are not many of these examples documented in the English literature as not enough research has been done in these areas in the west. Such a text will help practitioners of both disciplines to be aware of the problems of unusual adverse effects in patient responses after drug treatments that may be due to CHM and OM interactions. Examples cited in the present texts are those translated from Chinese texts originated from literature and clinical journals available in China.

Readers who have prior knowledge of pharmacology and therapeutics of OM and treatment using CHM products may find the topics included in the text appropriate to their practice. The section on basic principles may well be too brief for newcomers to the field. Accordingly, references are given for both general and specific topics in each chapter. Practitioners are encouraged to keep records of observations made during their practice on incidents of interactions and make them available to their clinics for record purposes. It is hoped that such observations can be collected for further assessment and research for their clinical significance. As this is a growing and important field in patient care when both OM and CHM medications are used, the professions should establish some form of reporting system in a similar manner as the 'Yellow Card' scheme in the UK or 'Blue Card' system in Australia for reporting OM interactions and adverse effects. It is suggested that practitioners in appropriate academic or professional institutes, organisations, or universities should keep records of incidents of herb-drug interactions. Once a database has been established health authorities can be persuaded to fund assessment and validation of the observed interactions between CHM and OM medications.

The text is divided into four sections. Section One gives accounts of general principles and is subdivided into five chapters. Chapter One describes different categories of drug interactions (DIs), definitions, diversities and differences between CHM and OM medications and literature availability and interpretation of DIs. Chapters Two and Three review briefly concepts of pharmacokinetics and pharmacodynamics and mechanisms of orthodox DIs respectively. Chapters Four and Five describe concisely CHM concepts of using herbs and CHM prescriptions respectively. Section Two has two chapters (six and seven). Chapter Six describes observations of the use of CHM products and OM drugs in the east and the west and Chapter Seven is divided into two parts, in which Part 1 summarises examples leading to beneficial effects and Part 2 deals with interactions leading to adverse effects. Section Three attempts to introduce 'Training, Research and Documentation' in which Chapter Eight emphasises the importance of 'training professionals qualified in both OM and TCM practice' and Chapter Nine proposes areas for 'Research and Documentation'. The final section consists of three appendices which list commonly used CHM herbs classified according to TCM concepts (Appendix 1), the same but classified according to published pharmacological actions (Appendix 2) and the commonly available ready-made CHM products from TCM prescriptions (Appendix 3). Each chapter has its own references. The book will help the following health professionals in their practices: TCM and OM practitioners who prescribe CHM products, community pharmacists and health care professionals who stock CHM medications, hospital pharmacists and toxicological units staff, medical herbalists, undergraduates and postgraduates who are studying TCM as a new discipline and researchers in the CHM fields will find this book useful.

Kelvin Chan
Lily Cheung

ACKNOWLEDGEMENTS

Before writing this text quite a lot of preliminary groundwork has been involved. We are grateful to various colleagues in the organisations and institutes concerning traditional Chinese medicine (TCM) that Professor Chan visited in China, Japan, Hong Kong and Taiwan during his Churchill Fellowship in 1995/1996. They have provided valuable materials in different aspects of TCM, including; teaching, research and development, practice, and regulations on the use and manufacture of Chinese herbal medicinal products. Some of this information has been incorporated in appropriate sections of this text. We thank Mr Liu for his help in compiling the tables in Chapter Seven and the Appendices.

One of us, Kelvin Chan, would like to acknowledge that he has spent a lot of spare time preparing and writing this book. This should have been spent with his wife, Gail, and children, Debra and Andrew.

Section One

General Principles

1. GENERAL CONSIDERATION OF ORTHODOX DRUGS, CHINESE HERBAL MEDICINAL (CHM) PRODUCTS AND TYPES OF DRUG INTERACTIONS

KELVIN CHAN

BENEFICIAL VERSUS UNDESIRABLE DRUG INTERACTIONS IN DRUG TREATMENT

It is advisable that polypharmacy should be avoided in order to prevent the occurrence of drug interactions. In certain circumstances, it is necessary that several drugs are included for treatment of some diseases. The practitioners should have a good grasp of the pharmacology of drugs when the treatment involves a multiple drug regimen. In general, many of the interactions that may occur in OM practice involving combinations of orthodox medications are harmless and sometimes beneficial if the purpose of combination is known. For example, the interaction between a local anaesthetic and vasoconstrictors (adrenaline) for inducing local anaesthesia in dental treatment; in combination the vasoconstrictor reduces tissue perfusion and restricts the absorption of local anaesthetic from the site of injection. A number of drug interactions, however, can be hazardous or harmful. It is essential to take a thorough drug history before prescribing, as interactions may occur with already prescribed drugs or self-medication of other remedies.

There are examples that self-medication is commonplace among patients of certain ethnic groups. The recent popularity of patients seeking medical treatment from traditional Chinese medicine (TCM) practitioners has revealed the need of assessing the possibility of interactions between orthodox medicinal (OM) and Chinese herbal medicine (CHM) products. Moreover in some Chinese communities, self-medication with CHM products is not uncommon for their belief that these products are good tonic food for recuperation after surgery or major operations in hospitals.

Complications arise when one considers the differences between the practice of OM and CHM both in diagnosis and in treatment approaches. Nevertheless it is possible to consider and assess the pharmacological and therapeutic actions and properties of OM medications and CHM products in order to make a scientific assessment of the likelihood of interactions. In the Chinese literature there are many clinical examples of interactions cited as important observations. The knowledge of pharmacological and therapeutic actions of OM and CHM products is extremely important for assessment purposes. The following texts will be arranged to give a systematic picture on these issues and to help practitioners and health-care professionals to take up an interest of the subject and be vigilant in their practice and research on the topics.

SOME DEFINITIONS

Drugs are chemically pure substances which when administered into the body produce pharmacological effects (therapeutic and side effects); the consequences of these may alleviate illnesses, help diagnosis or prevent disorders.

Medicines are formulated preparations containing active ingredients.

Chinese herbal medicinal (CHM) products or generally known as Chinese materia medica are used for treatment of diseases, or as tonics, and substances for prevention of illnesses according to traditional Chinese medicine (TCM) diagnosis and therapeutics. The majority of CHM come from plant sources, though some are of mineral or animal origin, hence they are collectively known as Chinese herbs. Most Chinese herbs are prescribed or taken as a mixture of several herbs in aqueous decoctions. Some are presented as CHM ready-made products of various dosage forms.

Drug Interactions (DIs) are phenomena during drug therapy when the pharmacological or therapeutic actions of a drug are altered by the co-administration of other drugs or substances. The consequence can be either an exaggeration of pharmacological or toxic effects or a diminished efficacy of drug treatment. In both cases, such interactions may lead to therapeutic failure and endanger patients' conditions. The relevance of drug interactions depends on how clinically significant is the therapeutic outcome. Thus we can consider different categories of drug interactions.

CATEGORIES OF DRUG INTERACTIONS

The classification of DIs into different categories (based on Evaluation of Drug Interaction, 3rd Edition, Shinn, AF, Shrewsbury RP) depends on ongoing research and development relating to clinical experience and experimental findings in drug use. The practitioner is cautioned to consult carefully information available for the medicines prior to their administration for added precautions or warnings.

(1) **Highly clinically significant** — those are of great potential harm to the patient, are predictable or occur frequently and well documented.
(2) **Moderately clinically significant** — those are of moderate potential harm to the patient, less predictable or occur less frequently or lack complete documentation.
(3) **Minimally clinically significant** — those are of little potential harm to the patient, have variable predictability or occur infrequently, are not documented.
(4) **Not clinically significant** — those could occur with documentation based on theoretical ground or resulting effects with very little significance or no adverse effects.

AVAILABILITY OF ORIGINAL LITERATURE AND INTERPRETATION ON INCIDENTS OF DRUG INTERACTIONS

It is reported in literature that the therapeutic or toxic effects of a drug, relatively safe when used alone, can be greatly affected by interactions with other drugs, food, environmental substances (e.g. hydrocarbons from cigarette smoking or pesticides etc.) or endogenous substances (hormones, neuro-transmitters and vitamins). Serious crises (death) have been reported and many less dramatic but clinically significant are often overlooked and not repeated. Many reports on potential DIs and long lists of such interactions have been compiled. But some of these reports are based on insufficient data, questionable protocols, insufficient patients and animal data, therefore, this will make interpretation difficult. DIs can occur outside or inside the body. Literature on the in vivo DIs and the adverse (mostly) or beneficial (seldom) clinical events that follow is plentiful. Fewer well reported are the in vitro DIs. In vitro DIs can occur during the formulation of the drug, during the addition of drugs to existing intravenous fluids, or during storage of active drugs in plastic containers (due to adsorption). In vivo DIs result in either drug toxicity or drug inefficiency while in vitro DIs often result in reduced bioavailability (or reduced drug efficacy).

Estimating how frequent DIs that have contributed to increased toxicity or decreased efficacy is not easy. It is possible to relate a significant increase in adverse effects to the use of multiple drug therapy. Several basic problems have been identified in interpreting and using existing literature information to reduce the incidence and severity of DIs:

(1) **Evaluate** the validity and clinical significance of the reported DIs.
(2) **Detect and prevent** DIs that are known to cause potential hazard.
(3) **Determine** the significance of a reported DI in a specific patient.
(4) **Recognise** previously unreported interactions.

Most clinically significant DIs are detected by the qualitative observation during treatment with several drugs concurrently. The mechanisms involved can be investigated by quantitative measurements using subsequent definitive studies. These include (a) pharmacological or therapeutic response that can be quantitated, e.g. prothrombin times, serum glucose levels, blood pressure, ECG, and (b) time course of plasma / serum concentrations of drugs and metabolites or their changes at steady state concentrations.

These informations are reported as observations in journals. Reliable literature on DIs can be found in several drug interaction reference books (refer to the list of General References). These also give references to original literature, apart from categories of DIs.

However, very little information, in English, is available for the DIs between Chinese herbal medicinal (CHM) products and orthodox drugs. An effort is needed to translate coordinate and report with careful interpretation on literature available. It is essential to research into the mechanisms of DI between these two groups of medications when they are used together intentionally, unknowingly and unintentionally.

DIVERSITIES OF POTENT THERAPEUTIC AGENTS

Great diversities in chemical structures, physico-chemical properties with quite different pharmacological effects exist among numerous compounds that are used as therapeutic agents. When these agents are concurrently administered, they may interact in a number of ways. It is useful to note this information well so that DIs can be avoided or minimised,

Table 1.1 Five physico-chemical groups of drugs

Groups	Characteristics	Examples
Water-soluble and highly polar drugs	Highly ionised, strong acids with pka $\cong$ 0; 100% ionised in the body: Drugs with multiple polar groups	Drug conjugates, heparin, mannitol, streptomycin, kanamycin, and other aminoglycoside antibiotics
	Highly ionised, strong bases with pka $\cong$ 14; 100% ionised in the body: Mono-onium compounds	Edrophonium, neostigmine, pyridostigmine
	Di-onium compounds	Suxamethonium, gallamine triethiodide
Drugs with intermediate polarity	Not as strongly polar and water soluble as in Group 1	digoxin, tetracycline
Lipid soluble and non-polar agents many examples	slightly acidic	Barbiturates, phenytoin, meprobamate; all depress CNS activities.
	virtually neutral	Digitoxin, chloral hydrate, ether, ethanol
	slightly basic	Theophylline, acetanilide
Weakly acidic drugs with pka 2 to 8 many examples	similar ADME characteristics with diverse modes of pharmacological profiles	Acetylsalicyclic acid, indomethacin, and most NSAID analgesics; Warfarin and related anticoagulants; Penicillins and related antibiotics; Sulphonamides, and related compounds such as acetazolamide diuretics; Sulphonylurea anti-diabetic: tolbutamide
Weakly basic drugs with pka 6–12 many examples	Their unionised moieties are lipid soluble and have similar ADME modes with diversified pharmacological actions. EXAMPLES include: morphine, pethidine and their related narcotic analgesics; bupivacaine and related local anaesthetics; lignocaine, morizicine anti-arrhythmics; atropine, hyoscine and related anti-cholinergics; adrenaline, isoprenaline, amphetamine, ephedrine and related sympathomimetics; propranolol and related β-adrenergic blockers; diazepam and related anti-anxiety agents; chlorpromazine and related neuroleptics, imipramine and related anti-depressives; chlorpheniramine and related anti-histamines	

because experimental findings and clinical experience have shown that the great majority of DIs occur by a small number of basic mechanisms.

(1) **Physico-chemical properties of drugs** — All clinically used orthodox drugs can be broadly classified into 5 physico-chemical groups (Table 1.1) with different pharmacological actions. This classification is based on their characteristic patterns of drug disposition in the body. The two major properties of a drug molecule that determine

its fate of disposition are the degree of ionization (pKa) and the lipid solubility of the unionized moiety. The two properties also determine the access of the molecule to the site of actions. The potency, however, depends on how the molecule fits into receptors. This depends on many other factors that relate structure-activity of the drug.

(2) **Pharmacological/Therapeutic/Adverse effects** — The development of a new chemical into a clinically accepted drug requires painstaking screening in pre-clinical stages for pharmacological and toxicological effects. The initial therapeutic effects can only be observed when the drug is at the early clinical trial stages. An ideal drug should have specific therapeutic action without side effects. However, invariably most drugs do produce side effects. Patients can tolerate some of these and those drugs with severe adverse effects would eventually be withdrawn if these side effects were life threatening. Thus untoward reactions to drugs can be the results of the following reasons:

(a) *Allergy (or hypersensitivity) to drugs* — is an immune response occurs in an individual who has been prior-exposed to the drugs.

(b) *Intolerance to a given drug* occurs when side effects appear at doses tolerated by most individuals e.g. some elderly patients cannot tolerate new non-steroidal anti-inflammatory drugs that have been withdrawn from medical use after 10 years in the market.

(c) *Idiosyncratic response to drugs* from individuals who are deficient in drug metabolism capacity e.g. patients deficient in glucose-6-phosphate dehydrogenase develop haemolytic anaemia after exposure to primaquine.

(d) *Adverse drug interactions* — these occur consequential to co-administration of two or more drugs together.

(3) **A Comparison of Orthodox Drugs and Chinese Medicinal Herbs (CMH) and Products.**

Tables 1.2. and 1.3. summarise the differences between the physico-chemical and biological properties of the two categories respectively. It is clearly seen that very little common characteristics can be found from these two vastly different groups. Orthodox drugs are pure single compounds while each CMH product may contain many chemical entities not defined. The chemical contents are far more complicated when several

Table 1.2 Differences between orthodox drugs and TCM herbs (Physico-Chemical Characteristics)

Properties	Orthodox drugs*	TCM herbs**
Active ingredients	Known	Very often unknown
Pure compound available	Yes	Rarely
Accessible for analysis	Yes	Complex/Difficult
Raw materials available	Dependable	Limited/exhaustible
Quality of the raw materials	Good	Variable
Standardisation	Easy	Difficult/achievable
Stability	Achievable	Difficult/achievable

*Orthodox drugs refer to chemically defined and established drugs.
**TCM herbs refer to either single herb or combination of several herbs in one prescription.
(Adopted from K. Chan, Progress in traditional Chinese medicine, TiPs June 1995; Vol. 16, 182—187).

Table 1.3 Differences between orthodox drugs and TCM herbs (Biological Characteristics)

Properties	Orthodox drugs*	TCM herbs**
Mechanism of actions	Known in most cases	Often unknown
Toxicology tests from pre-clinical screening	Mandatory	Most often not available; been used in clinical practice
Empirical data	Often meaningless	Important from cumulative clinical experience
Therapeutic experience over extended periods	No; in particular for recently developed drugs	Well-known prescriptions been used over generations
Adverse effects	Present	Rare from well used herbs or prescriptions
Tolerance	Limited	Usually very good
Therapeutic window	Usually potent (narrow)	Wide
Suitability for chronic use	Usually not yet tested/limited	Often well tested
Placebo controls	Easy	Difficult
Controlled Clinical trials and adequate statistical evaluation	Usually mandatory	Usually cases-studies

*Orthodox drugs refer to chemically defined established drugs.
**TCM herbs refer to either single herb or combination of several herbs in one prescription.
(Adopted from K. Chan, Progress in traditional Chinese medicine, TiPs June 1995; Vol. 16, 182–187).

herbs are included in a CMH prescription for treatment. The mechanisms of action are clearly defined for synthetic drugs whilst that of CMH products are not understood from orthodox medicine's view point even though CMH herbs are used according to the traditional Chinese medicine principles and practice. The choice and combination of CMH in a Chinese medicine prescription is a reflection of the deficiency and imbalance present in the body that is diagnosed and rectified by the herbs. More information on the scientific principles of using Chinese medicinal herbs and their combinations will be presented in later chapters.

2. REVIEW ON THE PRINCIPLES OF PHARMACOKINETICS AND PHARMACODYNAMICS

KELVIN CHAN

INTRODUCTION

In order to appreciate how a drug works it is essential that the principles behind drug disposition and pharmacokinetics should be understood. Drug disposition is a comprehensive term that includes the processes of absorption, distribution, metabolism and excretion (ADME) of the drug molecules after administration of the medicine into the body. It is possible from the physico-chemical characteristics of a drug molecule one can make valid predictions about its fate in the body. An accurate knowledge of ADME of a drug is of critical importance in clinical medicine in drug therapy, pharmacy and toxicology.

CONCEPTS OF DRUG DISPOSITION

Absorption refers to the entry of drug molecules into the blood via the mucous membranes of the alimentary (orally) or respiratory tracts (by inhalation) or from the skin (transdermally) or from the sites of injection (intramuscularly or subcutaneously). *Distribution* is defined as the movement of drug molecules between the water and lipid and protein constituents or other tissues of the body. *Metabolism* is involved with the endogenous processes of altering of the structure of the drug molecule, also known as biotransformation; as a means of detoxification (in most cases) or activation (in rare cases). In some cases, the consequence is production of toxic metabolites. The majority of drug metabolism takes place in the liver. *Excretion* is the removal of the original drug molecule and its metabolites from the body via mainly the kidneys and other routes such as the bile, the breath and the skin.

   Drug Metabolism or biotransformation has two main important consequences on the drug molecule. Firstly the lipid soluble drug is made more hydrophilic or polar (hence, more water soluble) thus hastening the excretion of its metabolite by the kidneys because the less lipid-soluble metabolite is not readily reabsorbed from the renal tubules. Secondly the metabolites are usually less active than the original drug but sometimes are equally or more active than the parent molecule. In some cases the metabolites can be toxic. Certain pro-drugs, as purposely designed, become only active after biotransformation. The liver is the main site of enzyme systems that are responsible for drug metabolism, but the gastrointestinal tract (GI tract), lungs and kidneys have considerable enzyme activities. Orally given drugs, absorbed from the small intestine directly via the portal system to the liver, are extensively metabolised. This is referred to as *first-pass metabolism* indicating that metabolism may also occur in the GI tract. Hence the bioavailability, F, of orally

9

absorbed drugs, if they are subject to extensive drug metabolism, is always lower than intravenously administered (F = 1). These drugs are only effective when given parenterally. The drug metabolising enzyme systems in the liver are responsible for both *Phase I and Phase II reactions*. *Phase I reactions* involve the biotransformation of a drug to a more polar metabolite(s) by introducing or unmasking a functional group(s) such as -COOH, -OH, $-NH_2$, $-SH_2$, involving enzymatic reactions such as oxidation (most common one), reduction, and hydrolysis. Many of these enzymes are located on the smooth endoplasmic reticulum (SER) which are identified as small vesicles; when the SER is homogenised and after differential centrifugation the preparation is known as the liver microsomal enzyme system. This system is better known as the *cytochrome P-450* mixed function oxidase system, which as a group of enzymes, has very low substrate specificity as many different drugs can be oxidised. As a requirement, microsomal oxidation in the liver involves the co-factor, NADPH, oxygen and two other co-enzymes (NADPH-cytochrome P-450 reductase and cytochrome P-450 which acts as a terminal oxidase). Due to the advancement of biotechnological separation, cytochrome P-450 has been confirmed as a family of different iso-enzymes, each of which has its own specificity for certain chemical groups and is characteristically linked to certain chromosomal localisation of the ancestral gene. Thus there is variability of the capacity in drug metabolism; hence, variability in drug responses among different individuals and different ethnic groups. The study of how genetic determinants affect drug response is known as *Pharmacogenetics*.

Such observations have important consequence on individual susceptibility to adverse effects due to drug treatment. About 5% of the Caucasian population are poor hydroxylators and show exaggerated and prolonged responses to anti-hypertensive drugs such as metoprolol and propranolol. Readers are referred to the textbook by Price Evans (1996) for detail information. Other *Phase I reactions* such as reductions and hydrolyses are also non-specific. *Phase II reactions* in the liver involve conjugation of the drug or Phase I metabolites with endogenous compounds such as glycine or other amino acids, glucuronic acid, sulphate ions. The resulting conjugates are often less active than the parent drug and Phase I metabolites. This process makes the drug molecules more polar and water-soluble enabling rapid excretion by the kidneys. During Phase II metabolism if the endogenous substance is depleted due to the formation of excessive toxic or reactive Phase I metabolites, drug toxicity will occur. Paracetamol, a widely self-medicated weak analgesic normally eliminated by glucuronidation and sulphation, when ingested with high dose (over 15g or 30 paracetamol 500mg tablets), will produce reactive metabolite when the conjugation paths are saturated. This reactive intermediate, normally conjugated by glutathione whose store becomes depleted during overdose, accumulates and reacts with hepatocyte causing liver necrosis. N-acetylcysteine that provides the -SH group for conjugating the reactive metabolite is used as an anti-dote in paracetamol poisoning due to overdose.

Renal Excretion is the ultimate elimination process for most drugs and metabolites. The rate of their renal elimination depends on the renal blood flow, protein-binding capacity and the physico-chemical properties of the molecules. In a healthy individual the renal excretion of inulin, which is not protein-bound and is not re-absorbed from the renal tubule, is 120ml per minute (i.e. 120ml of blood is cleared of inulin in 1 minute) which is a measure of the filtration rate and is a reflection of the renal function of the healthy individual. Lipid soluble drugs after filtration into the renal tubules are often re-absorbed back to the blood stream depending on their ionisation constants (pKa values). Thus metabolism aids renal excretion as it renders drugs more polar and water-soluble. The ionisation of weak acids and bases depends on the pH of the tubular fluid. Alteration of the urinary pH can help elimination of weak acids or bases. Sodium bicarbonate administration alkalinises urinary pH and helps elimination of weak acids such as aspirin which exists mostly as ionised moiety and is less lipid soluble in alkaline urine. Acid urine conditions help elimination of amphetamine, a weak base.

Extrarenal excretion includes excretion via the lungs and the skin through the sweat (if the drug molecules are relatively small), the bile, the milk, the saliva and through the placenta. These processes have their own important position in relation to drug disposition. Drugs, which are concentrated into the bile, are secreted into the small intestine where they may be re-absorbed, thus creating an entero-hepatic circulation that may increase the persistence of a drug in the body. Biliary excretion often involves drugs and conjugates of metabolites with relatively larger molecules and higher molecular weights. Transport of drugs into the milk and through the placenta obviously requires extra attention during drug treatment for the patients. Excretion of drugs via the saliva is sometimes used as a non-invasive monitoring of concentration of drugs in the body. Physico-chemical properties of drug molecules and physiological factors play an important part in determining the extent that drugs can be eliminated via these extra renal routes.

In conclusion, the importance of ADME processes is that they collectively determine the concentration of drug molecules at the site of drug action (or the receptor) and thus influencing pharmacologic effects. Therefore, two significant aspects are involved after drug administration: Influence of the body on the drug (the ADME) and the influence of the drug on the body to produce the required pharmacologic response (the pharmacodynamic effects). If ADME are ignored the patient may suffer from the following consequences: (a) Toxic drugs may accumulate in the body to produce harmful or even fatal effects, (b) Useful drugs may be without effects, as too low a dose to achieve therapeutic level or the patient does not take the dose and (c) Inter-subject variations in some or all of the ADME processes may be influenced by in disease states such as renal or hepatic insufficiency. Figure 1 illustrates the fate of a reversibly acting drug in the body after administration. Sufficiently lipid soluble drugs, after orally absorbed, are rapidly distributed throughout the body. Many drugs are loosely bound to plasma proteins, in particular albumin, in equilibrium forming between the bound and free drug in the plasma. Drugs that are highly protein bound are confined to the vascular system and are not able to exert their pharmacological actions. Figure 1 also indicates the likely sites of drug interactions in the body after co-administration of other medications. It is obvious that the ADME processes and its effects at the site of the primary drug can be affected by the interacting medications at these sites.

PRINCIPLES OF PHARMACOKINETICS

Pharmacokinetics describes how the body handles drug molecules with reference to time. It is an applied approach that gives the mathematical description of how drug concentration and activity changes with time after administration of the drug to the body. This include

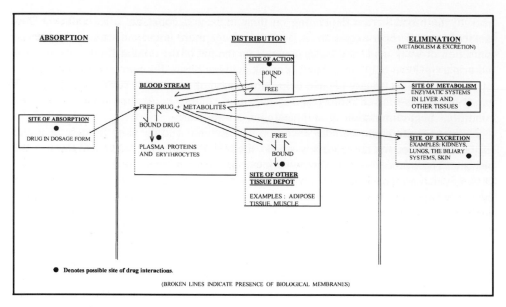

Figure 1   The fate of a reversely acting drug in the body.

the kinetics of absorption, distribution, metabolism and other elimination (i.e. the ADME) of the drug. The purpose of pharmacokinetics is to study the time course of the amounts of drug and its metabolites in the blood/plasma, different tissues and excreta and to construct mathematical models that can interpret accurately observed data. The application of these data to dosage design will help correct use of medications.

Derivation of Pharmacokinetic Parameters

In the simplest situation after intravenous administration the drug enters the blood and is rapidly distributed to various tissues within the body. From a series venous blood sample the decrease in plasma concentrations of the drug with time can be measured and followed graphically. For most drugs the plasma concentration falls rapidly at the initial phase and then the rate of decline progressively decreases in an exponential manner. The plasma concentration time-curve follows an exponential decline meaning that at any given time a constant fraction of the drug present is eliminated in unit time. This exponential elimination of the drug is governed by the first order rate (in most cases) elimination processes taking places via the urine by glomerular filtration, metabolism in the liver, uptake by the liver with subsequent elimination in the bile and other organs of the body. If any enzyme responsible for drug metabolism becomes saturated, the elimination kinetics becomes zero order meaning that the elimination rate proceeds at a constant rate and is unaffected any increase in concentrations of the drug. Examples of drugs behaving in this manner are ethanol and phenytoin. Similarly, if the renal elimination capacity of the drug is affected by active competition of another the elimination will not follow first order kinetics.

Mathematically the fate of the drug after reaching the circulation can be represented by measuring the elimination half life ($T_{1/2}$) of the drug from the circulation which is defined as the time taken for the drug concentration in the blood to fall by half of its original value. Measurement of the $T_{1/2}$ allows determination of the elimination rate constant (K_{el}) from the expression: $K_{el} = 0.693/T$. By definition K_{el} is the fraction of the drug present at any time that would be eliminated in unit time assuming linear (first order) kinetics is operating. Thus when $K_{el} = 0.05$ minute^{-1} it means that 5% of the drug present is eliminated in 1 minute. The value of $C°$, initial apparent drug concentration, can be determined graphically. The **APPARENT VOLUME OF DISTRIBUTION**, V_d, is a valuable parameter that describes how widely the drug is distributed in the body. It can be derived from the expression: $V_d = DOSE/C°$, when the intravenous **DOSE** and the apparent initial drug concentration are known. A value of $V_d < 5$ to 6 litres suggests that the drug is mainly retained within the vascular compartment. A value < 15 litres implies the drug is restricted to the extravascular fluid, but any values of $V_d > 15$ litres indicate wide distribution throughout the total body water with penetration to other tissues. V_d is important for determination of **CLEARANCE, CL** (in litres per unit time) which is required for calculation of the dosage of the drug. Clearance is an important concept as it is the volume of the blood or plasma cleared of drug in unit time and can be derived from the expression: $CLp = V_d \times K_{el}$. Clearance is the sum of individual clearance values from various organs. Thus, $CLp = CLm + Clr$ refers to the total plasma clearance is the sum of metabolism clearance and renal clearance. The dosing regimen of a drug is often calculated by referring to the steady state drug concentration, **Cpss**, at a known therapeutic range. A steady state is only reached when the rate of drug entering the systemic circulation (**dosing rate = Clp × Cpss**) equals to the rate of elimination. The expression: **F × DOSE /dosing interval = Clp × Cpss** is often used for calculating dosage after oral administration where **F is the bioavailability** of the drug which describes the proportion of administered drug reaching the systemic circulation. Its value is 100% after intravenous dose (F = 1). Drugs are usually given orally and the fraction of the dose reaching the circulation varies with various drugs and different patients.

PRINCIPLES OF PHARMACODYNAMICS

Pharmacodynamics describes how drugs produce effects on the body. The simplest concept one can follow is to consider that the normal functions of the body probably depend on a series of biochemical and physiological processes that are controlled and mediated by endogenous substances or chemical compounds that are produced by the body at regular intervals with defined quantities. These endogenous substances can be transmitters, enzymes, and hormones which can be simple amino acids, chemical compounds, small molecules of proteins, or peptides.

They can act as agonists or antagonists on established receptors, enzymes or transport processes. Diseases that occur probably due to abnormalities arise from biochemical or physiological malfunction of the body. Drugs are administered to rectify these malfunctions. They can be replacement or act as agonists or antagonists of the endogenous substances.

Mechanisms of Drug Action

A drug can produce its pharmacological effects by acting on receptors, enzymes, and transport processes. Only a few drugs, such as general anaesthetics and osmotic diuretics, act by *non-specific drug action*, by virtue of their physico-chemical properties. Some drugs may act as false transmitters or inhibitors for certain transport processes or enzymes. Most drugs produce their effects by acting on specific receptors that are protein molecules located in the cell membrane. These receptors normally respond to endogenous chemicals, either synaptic transmitters or hormones in the body.

Receptors are protein molecules that are normally activated by transmitters or hormones. *Transmitters* are endogenously synthesised chemicals released from nerve terminals that diffuse across the synaptic cleft and bind to the receptor. For example acetylcholine (the transmitter involved in the autonomic nervous system) released from motor nerve endings activates the receptors in skeletal muscle initiating a sequence of events that leads to the contraction of the muscle. Drugs, with closely related structures and characteristics to the transmitters, which activate the receptors and produce a response are referred to as *Agonists*. Some drugs are *antagonists* that do not activate but fit in well on the receptor thus reducing the probability of the transmitter acting on the receptor hence blocking agonist action. In some cases the activation of receptors by an agonist or hormone is coupled to some biochemical and physiological responses by transduction that often involve molecules called second messengers. The interaction between a drug and the binding site of the receptor depends on how well fit the linking of the two is. The better the fit and the greater the non-covalent bonds (in reversibly acting mechanism only, irreversible binding occurs by covalent binding) will result stronger and higher *affinity* of the drug molecule for the receptor. Ideally the drug should possess the *specificity* to bind one particular type of receptor; but no drug is completely specific. However, through pharmaceutical research and development and the application of quantitative structure activity relationship (QSAR) screening, many drugs available in the market have certain relative *selectivity* acting on one type of receptor. This is to minimise actions on other receptors hence side effects. In general, drugs are administered to produce a therapeutic effect but they often produce unwanted adverse effects. Moreover if the receptor involved is present in many tissues the drug will cause predictable adverse actions. Atropine, an antagonist of acetylcholine, blocks the acetylcholine receptors that are present in the brain, the eye, skin and the viscera. For whatever therapeutic reason atropine is given, it is likely to cause dry mouth, blurred vision, constipation and urinary retention.

Enzymes are catalytic proteins that help to increase the rate of chemical reactions in the body. They also function as regulators for controlling the duration of actions of endogenous transmitters. Drugs can be inhibitors of these enzymatic reactions by acting on the enzymes. Similar concepts on specificity and selectivity apply for drugs used as enzyme inhibitors. Drugs, such as neostigmine, that inhibit cholinesterases and enhance the action of acetylcholine are administered to reverse the action of neuromuscular blocking agents such as tubocurarine. Thiazides are weak carbonic anhydrase inhibitors used for treatment of hypertension and mild heart failure due to their mild diuretic effects by inhibiting the catalysis of carbon dioxide with increase in the excretion of bicarbonate and sodium ions and water. Phenelzine, a nonselective and irreversible monoamine oxidase inhibitor (MAOI), is used as the last choice in the treatment of atypical depressive and phobic anxiety states. Irreversible MAOIs possess many adverse effects such as postural hypotension, dizziness, anticholinergic effects and interactions with other food and drugs, due to their nonselectivity. This is because the normal functions of monoamine oxidase reactions are also affected due to presence of phenelzine.

Second messengers are endogenous chemicals whose intracellular concentration increase in most instants and rarely decrease when the receptors are activated by agonists that trigger processes that lead to cellular responses. Examples of these second messengers are calcium ions, cyclic adenosine monophosphate (cAMP), diacylglycerol (DG) and inosito-1, 4, 5-triphosphate (IP_3). These second messengers have significant roles to keep neuro-transmission and maintain other biochemical and physiological functions of the body. Drugs that interfere with these processes can inevitably cause unwanted side effects unless they have definite selectivity and specificity in their actions.

REFERENCES

The reference list below gives some typical texts for readers' information on general pharmacology and concepts of drug disposition, pharmacokinetics and pharmacodynamics.

Gibaldi, M. and Perrier, D (1982) *Pharmacokinetics*. In: *Drugs and the Pharmaceutical sciences,* **Vol. 15**, Marcel Dekker, New York and Basle.

Hardman, J.G., Limbird, L.E., Molinoff, P, B., Ruddon, R.W. and Gilman, A.G. (1996) *Goodman & Gilman's The Pharmacoloigcal Basis of Therapeutics*, Ninth Edition, MaGraw-Hill, International Edition.

Katzung, B.G. (1995) *Basic and Clinical Pharmacology*, 9th Edition, Appleton & Lange, International Edition.

Laurence, D. R., Bennett, P.N. and Brown, M.J. (1997) *Clinical Pharmacology*, 8th edition, Churchill Livingston, International Edition.

Neal, M.J. (1993) *Medical Pharmacology at a Glance*, 2nd Edition, Blackwell Scientific Publication, Oxford.

3. MECHANISMS OF DRUG INTERACTIONS

KELVIN CHAN

IN VITRO DRUG INCOMPATIBILITY

It is important to appreciate that **Drug Incompatibility** occurs in vitro before administration to patients when two or more drugs are mixed together. This may be due to reactions or antagonistic changes in pharmaceutical formulations, denoting an inability to mixing the drugs together. These in vitro drug interactions can occur during formulation of an active drug ingredient with other excipients, in the process of adding drugs to existing formulation, and during the storage of formulated drugs in plastic syringes or containers. The consequences are often related to reduction in bioavailability or reduced drug efficacy during storage and resulting in therapeutic failure.

Incompatibility in Formulated Medicines often occurs due to presence of certain excipients or pharmaceutical adjuvant other than the active drug itself. These substances facilitate formulation into a stable, uniform, acceptable medicine with the required bioavailability and release characteristics. Examples of excipients include: aerosol propellants, antioxidants, binders, colours, disintegrants, fillers, flavours, lubricants, preservatives, solubilisers, solvents, surfactants, suspending agents, sweeteners and thickeners. They, in combinations with the active drug, make up the bulk of an oral solid dosage form. Classical examples of formulation problems are: Phenytoin intoxication (Tyrer, 1970) broke out in Australia due to change in capsule filler from calcium sulphate to lactose. Increase in dissolution rate leading to increased bioavailability and toxicity in patients who took the new formulated phenytoin tablets. Rifampicin absorption was impaired by p-amino-salicylic acid (PAS), due to presence of bentonite in the PAS granules, thus, causing reduced efficacy of anti-TB treatment. Bioavailability problems with digoxin (Lanoxin) tablets were related to reduced particle size of digoxin. Increased bioavailability of the new formulation led to overdigitalisation of previously stabilised patients.

Incompatibility due to Additives to Intravenous Fluids: is related to incompatibility or unstableness of the admixture that contain several drugs in the intravenous solution which are in stable form on their own. Degradation of the active ingredients may occur because pH of the solutions is dissimilar, solubility of the drugs may be altered. For example, soluble insulin injection should not be mixed with protamine zinc insulin in the same syringe as the soluble insulin will react with the excess zinc and protamine, thus reducing bioavailability of insulin. Materials of syringe or needle may interact with injection solution; e.g. doxorubicin HCl injection solution reacts with the aluminum hub of a syringe needle.

Interactions between Drug and Containers: have been reported for the sorption of drugs to IV fluid containers, delivery sets, syringes, filters or other plastic apparatus, indicating that the polyvinyl chloride (PVC) is the major offender. Drugs that are likely to be adsorbed to plastic materials are amiodarone, chlorethiazole, diazepam, insulin, isosorbide dinitrate, lignocaine, and vitamin A acetate. Some drugs alter the physical

17

appearance of plastic materials. For example, cyclopropane and volatile anaesthetics such as methoxyflurane partially solubilises PVC plastics; paraldehyde solubilises polystyrene and styrene-acryl nitrile copolymer.

MECHANISMS OF DRUG INTERACTIONS

There are two possible types of drug-drug interactions: Pharmacokinetic interactions and pharmacodynamic interactions. The former can be defined as consequences in which one or several drugs alter the rate or extent of gastro-intestinal absorption, distribution, metabolism or excretion of another drug. The latter describe the consequences of increasing or decreasing drug therapeutic or toxic effects, at receptors, enzyme systems or transport systems that govern the normal biochemical or physiological functions of the body, when more than two or several drugs are acting on the same or related systems. The precise mechanisms in pharmacodynamic interactions may not be fully understood and predicted due probably to the complexity of interactions involved at molecular levels. However, pharmacokinetic interactions can be predicted and prevented when adequate scientific and practice evidence are recorded. Some complications in drug interactions will arise when inter-individual variability in response to drug effects or idiosyncratic responses to drug treatment are involved. Under these circumstances the mechanisms of drug interactions will be complex and require careful investigations. The general consequences of drug interactions are either an increase or a decrease in known therapeutic or toxic effects. Some drug-interactions are beneficial and have been used for years as a beneficial aid in drug therapy. In practice potentially lethal interactions such as potentiation of the actions of oral anticoagulants, hypoglycaemic agents and cytotoxic drugs etc are observed.

PHARMACOKINETIC DRUG INTERACTIONS

Interference with Drug Absorption

Theoretically the possibility for interactions are numerous because concomitant oral ingestion of drugs is by far the most common route of administration (up to 70%). But only a few interactions are known to be clinically significant. It is important to distinguish between drug absorption interactions which (a) increase or decrease the rate of absorption and (b) increase or decrease the extent or amount of drug absorbed.

The rate of drug absorption is usually not important for drugs with a long plasma half-life when given in multiple dose scheme to achieve a steady state concentration, e.g. psychotherapeutic agents (Chlorpromazine, imipramine) and anti-hypertensive drugs. In this case the amount of drug-absorbed determines the steady state concentration. But a decrease or delay rate of absorption is important in a clinical situation when a rapid onset of drug effect is desired. For example, in the relief of acute pain and insomnia rapid and high plasma concentration are desirable in a single dose of analgesic for headache or a hypnotic to induce sleep, respectively.

Considering the pharmacokinetic data of absorption of the affected drug can assess delayed absorption or decreased absorption due to the presence of another drug. The delayed absorption rate and the decrease in total area under the plasma or blood concentration time curve and the amount of urinary excretion of the unchanged drug and metabolites in relation to dose are good indications of interference at the absorption process.

Change in pH of GI Fluids: Antacids diminish the acidity of stomach content thus, decrease the absorption of acidic drugs such as salicylates, barbiturates, phenylbutazone by gastric walls; the absorption of basic drugs is enhanced (Not important in clinical practice). Gastric acid stimulants such as ethanol, meat extracts and amino acid lower gastric pH, thus enhancing absorption of acidic drugs (not important as most absorption takes place in the small intestine). To prevent the occurrence of the interaction it is advisable to administer other drugs at least 1/2 to 1 hour before antacid ingestion.

Motility of GI Tract: Anticholinergic drugs (atropine, belladonna preparation, propantheline) slow down gut movement, therefore diminish absorption of other drugs. For example, desipramine, a tricyclic antidepressive, delays the absorption of phenylbutazone. But some tricyclic antidepressants increase the absorption of dicoumarol anticoagulant that is poorly absorbed. Nortriptyline and imipramine increase bioavailability of dicourmarol. Metoclopramide significantly increases the rate of absorption of paracetamol due to an increase in gastric emptying rate, but the extent is not affected. Laxatives accelerate transport of bowel contents, therefore influence the enteral absorption of drugs and vitamins.

Binding Or Chelation Mechanisms: Metal ions in oral mixtures, containing Ca^{++}, Fe^{++}, Mg^{++}, Al^{+++}, reduce the total amount of tetracycline absorbed in man due to the formation of insoluble chelate or complexes between tetracycline and the metal ions. The interaction can be avoided if the drug preparations are given about 3 hours apart. Cholestyramine, an anionic resin used for treatment of hyperlipoproteinaemia, decreases the absorption of cardiac glycosides, oral anticoagulants (warfarin), calcium salts and bile acids. Para-amino salicylic acid tablets or granules impair the amount of rifampicin absorbed due to the adsorption of rifampicin by bentonite that is used as a major excipient in the preparation.

Other Mechanism: Beneficial drug interaction between local anaesthetic and adrenaline is used in dental practice as adrenaline constricts capillaries near the gum region and confines the local anaesthetic action of lignocaine whose systemic absorption if not checked can cause arrhythmia.

Interference with Drug Distribution

General Principles: Many drugs are extensively bound to plasma proteins or other tissues and it is generally accepted that only the unbound drug fraction is responsible for drug action. In vitro plasma protein binding studies have provided some evidence of displacement of a drug from its binding site(s) on albumin by other drug. But, in vitro extrapolation into in vivo situation is not always accurate. For example, the possible interaction between warfarin and indomethacin does not show potentiation of the hypoprothrombinaemic effect of warfarin after giving indomethacin, despite the fact that indomethacin displaces warfarin from its albumin binding sites in vitro. But, indomethacin causes gastric haemorrhage and ulceration and inhibits platelet aggregation. Oral anticoagulant may potentiate these undesirable effects.

Decreased in Plasma Protein Binding: In presence of other drugs, this is significant only for drugs which are highly protein-bound (> 90%) and which have a small apparent volume of distribution (App.Vol. Dist. $\cong 0.15$L/kg). This is because an increase in the fraction of unbound drug in plasma enables the free drug to diffuse into tissue with a consequent increase in App Vol. Dist. Generally a clinically significant DI may not be expected with highly bound drugs if their App Vol. Dist is large, i.e. only a small fraction of the drug in the body is found in plasma.

Displacement from Protein Binding Sites only has a continued and pronounced clinical effect when other mechanisms such as inhibition of drug metabolism are also involved.

Combination of different mechanisms: Phenylbutazone, oxyphenylbutazone and warfarin: That phenylbutazone potentiates the hypothrombinaemic effect of warfarin is often cited as a typical example of DI involving protein binding displacement. But other mechanism is also involved. Warfarin used in therapy consists of a racemic mixture of R&S enantiomeres (optically active). S-warfarin and R-warfarin are metabolically inactivated in the liver by formation of warfarin alcohol. The S-warfarin is several times more active than the R-warfarin. Phenylbutazone inhibits the metabolism of S-warfarin but induces the metabolism of R-warfarin. The net result is accumulations of S-warfarin therefore increase in anticoagulant effect. Clofibrate displaces dicoumarol from plasma protein binding sites thus increasing proportion of unbound fraction. It also inhibits dicoumarol metabolism.

Interference with Drug Metabolism

Drug Interactions Involving Stimulation of Drug Metabolism (Enzyme Induction)

General Principles: The intensity and duration of action of many drugs are related to the rate and extent of biotransformation to more polar and biologically inactive compounds (metabolites) by the drug metabolising enzyme system in the liver. (Refer to mechanisms involving metabolism and cytochrome P_{450}). The activity of these non-specific enzymes can be increased several fold by treatment with a large number of chemicals. This was first recognised by Conney and colleagues in 1956 when they showed an increase in N-demethylation of amino azo dye in rats pretreated with polycyclic hydrocarbon (3-methyl cholanthrene). In 1962, Remmer demonstrated during an investigation of drug tolerance that the loss of hypnotic potency of hexobarbitone in dogs following chronic dosing with the drug was due to an increase in the rate of oxidation and not to a change in receptor sensitivity.

There are two main types of enzyme induction: Phenobarbitone-induced and Polycyclic hydrocarbon-induced. Each type has its own characteristics. Possible inducers include commonly used drugs, insecticide, herbicides, polycyclic hydrocarbons (3-methyl cholanthrene), carcinogens, and natural compounds. In general, enzyme induction is associated with increased liver weight, increased production of microsomal protein and cytochrome P_{450} and other components in the endoplasmic reticulum.

Consequence of Enzyme Induction: These include, 1. Except in the rare instance where a drug metabolite is more active than the parent compounds, the administration of inducing drugs causes reduced pharmacological and toxic effects. 2. Enzyme induction may contribute to the development of drug tolerance. 3. Treatment with one inducing drug accelerates the metabolism of many other unrelated drugs. 4. The effect can persist for many days and weeks after the inhibiting drug is discontinued. 5. Difficulty arises in drug therapy if patients are exposed to industrial contaminants, e.g. the rate of metabolism of antipyrine is accelerated in workers exposed to indane dicophane.

Important Enzyme-Inducer in Clinical Use: Over 200 agents have been shown to be potent enzyme-inducers in animals but clinically important enzyme-inducers in man are not numerous. These are barbiturates, carbamazepine dichoral-phenazone, diphenylhydantoin, DDT insecticide, ethanol, griseofulvin, glutethimide, meprobamate, methaqualone, and phenylbutazone. These compounds have some common characteristics such as being lipid soluble in physiological pH, prolonged $t_{1/2}$ in plasma. Some have shorter $t_{1/2}$ only after repeated administration.

Beneficial Use of Enzyme Inducer: The application of such use should be dealt with caution. Induction can be useful clinically by administering phenobarbitone to accelerate the conjugation of bilirubin in neonatal hyperbilirubinaemia and familial unconjugated jaundice. Such use is now replaced by irradiating the jaundiced babies with ultra-violet light with suitable wavelength and caution. Induction does not occur rapidly to treat patients who have taken overdose of certain drugs. It is tempting to give an occasional dose of DDT to induce and thus protect patients who repeatedly make self-poisoning attempts.

Study Enzyme Induction in Man: 1. The activity of some of the enzyme in the liver microsomal enzyme system has been investigated in some patients undergoing 'open surgery liver biopsy'. However, this technique is difficult to perform. In general, direct measurement of this kind is rare to come by due to ethical permission. 2. The half-life of a test drug such as antipyrine can be measured as an indirect method. This is to establish the direct relationship between pre-induction antipyrine $t_{1/2}$ and the percentage decrease of antipyrine $t_{1/2}$ after treatment with the inducer. The longer the initial antipyrine $t_{1/2}$, the greater the reduction caused by phenobarbitone treatment. People with low metabolising activity are more inducible than others. A fall in steady state concentration of phenytoin is particularly marked in patients with high plasma level of phenytoin initially, after treatment with phenobarbitone. 3. The measurement of increased urinary excretion of endogenous substances such as D-glucaric acid, the metabolic by-product of 6 β-hydroxycortisol, is an indication of enzyme induction after ingestion of phenobarbitone or phenytoin in man.

Examples of Some Important and Documented DI Involving Enzyme Induction: 1. Barbituates decrease $t_{1/2}$ of oral anticoagulants by increasing their rate of metabolism with a consequent fall in the concentration of anticoagulant in the blood. Nearly all mostly used barbiturates increase metabolism of ethyl biscoumacetate, dicoumarol and warfarin. 2. Hepatotoxicity of paracetamol and haematotoxicity of phenacetin is enhanced by enzyme inducers. 3. Rifampicin shortens $t_{1/2}$ of tolbutamide and diminishes the effectiveness of oral contraceptives probably by increasing the rate of metabolism of the oestrogenic components. 4. Phenobarbitone and phenytoin are involved with important clinical observations. Steady state levels of phenytoin have been lowered in some patients by addition of phenobarbitone therapy. Phenytoin intoxication due to inhibition of parahydroxylation of phenytoin by phenobarbitone is also observed. These indicate both enzyme induction and inhibition metabolism of phenytoin due to phenobarbitone co-administration. Precise mechanism is unclear it may be due to the dose dependent kinetics of phenytoin as phenytoin metabolising enzymes are often saturated at serum concentration of phenytoin which lie within therapeutic range.

Drug Interactions Involving Inhibition of Drug Metabolism

General Principle: The metabolising activity of the liver microsomal enzyme system is not specific. Many drugs that are metabolised in the liver will, in principle, follow the same biotransformation pathways and will use the same microsomal enzyme system. In multiple drug therapy competition among such drugs for this system is expected. Therefore, metabolism of one drug may be inhibited by another drug given at the same time as both are competing for the same binding sites on the cytochrome P_{450}. In other cases, there is functional impairment of microsomal activity due to hepatotoxicity; inhibition produced by adrenaline, alloxan and PAS acid is associated with depletion of hepatic glycogen stores.

Consequence and Importance of Inhibition of Drug Metabolism: DIs due to inhibition of drug metabolising enzyme systems result in a rapid increase in effective drug concentration leading to exaggerated and prolonged response with an increased risk of toxicity. Enzyme inhibition may be clinically more important than induction of drug metabolism as the process is very much faster, but very little attention has been paid on this aspect. Clinical significance of interaction due to enzyme inhibition depends on the therapeutic ratio of the drug involved and the initial plasma concentrations of the acting drug before the inhibiting drug is given. For example, on chronic therapy of phenytoin, the inhibiting drug, chloramphenicol, produces phenytoin toxicity if the steady state phenytoin concentration is increased from 15μg/ml to 45μg/ml. However if the steady state level is increased from 5μg/ml to 15μg/ml no observable toxicity may be detected. The upper limit of plasma concentration for phenytoin toxicity to occur is around 20μg/ml.

Some Specific Enzyme Inhibitors: may also inhibit the liver microsomal enzyme system for metabolising other drugs. 1. Monoamine oxidase inhibitors (MAOI) such as isocarboxazid, pargyline, phenelzine, tranylopromine and trifluperazine produce their therapeutic effects by their ability to inhibit the enzyme, monoamine oxidase, which metabolises sympathomimetic amines in the tissue. These drugs also inhibit the metabolism of phenindione, barbiturates, tyramine and other endogenous amino acids involved in neuro-transmission. Consequence of such inhibition often results in hypertensive crisis. 2. Disulfiram is an inhibitor of the aldehyde dehydrogenase leading to accumulation of acetaldehyde and unpleasant symptoms when alcohol is ingested. The drug is used for treatment of alcoholism as a deterrent but also inhibits the metabolism of warfarin and phenytoin. Other drugs with disulfiram-like inhibition action are sulphonylureas, furazolidone and metronidazole. 3. Inhibitors of metabolic conjugation (glycine-conjugation,, glucuronidatio, sulphatation) such as aminobenzoic acid inhibit the glycine conjugation of salicylic acid and salicylamide blocks glucuronides formation of paracetamol and salicylic acid.

Examples of Some Important and Documented DI Involving Enzyme Inhibition: Several hundreds of inhibiting agents have been tested in animal experiments and not many inhibitors are identified in man. For example, SKF525A is a most widely used enzyme inhibitor in animal but does not appear to inhibit metabolism of other drugs in man. 1. Phenytoin's anti-convulsing activity and toxicity is potentiated by its decreased metabolism due to dicoumarol, disulfiram, isoniazid, para-amino-salicylic acid, warfarin and chloramphenicol. 2. Tolbutamide's activity is increased by its decreased metabolism due to aspirin, phenylbutazone, dicoumarol and sulphaphenazole. 3. Nortryptyline's activity is increased by its decreased biotransformation due to hydrocortisone and testosterone. 4. Warfarin's metabolism is inhibited by disulfiram with resulting increase in anticoagulant activity. 5. The activities of barbiturates, phenindione and tyramine are potentiated in presence of MAOIs that inhibit their metabolism.

Action to be Taken: If simultaneous administration is necessary the dose of the primary drugs should be reduced. It is also necessary to monitor carefully the polynomic effects and the plasma concentration of the primary drugs.

Interference with Drug Excretion

General Principles

Apart from inhalation anaesthetics most drugs and their metabolites are excreted through the kidneys. As blood passes through the glomeruli of the kidney tubules, drugs and other endogenous low molecular weight substances, except those that remain protein-bound, can leave the blood and filter through pores of the glomerular membrane. Large molecules such as the plasma proteins are, under normal conditions, retained in the blood. Along the tubules two independent active transport systems (one for acids and one for bases) remove drugs from the blood even if they are protein-bound and secrete then into the tubule. If molecules are either small and water soluble or large and lipid soluble they may also be reabsorbed into the blood by passive diffusion or active mechanisms similar to those concerned with secretion. Otherwise the drug is lost in the kidney filtrate. Therefore, it is possible for drug to interfere with these mechanisms to such an extent that the retention or loss of other drugs can be altered to provide a beneficial or a toxic effect.

Mechanisms for Interfering Renal Excretion: 1. During the re-absorption stage, changes in urinary pH will alter renal excretion of drugs. The renal clearance of basic drugs (pKa 7–11) is increased in acid urine and decreased in alkaline urine. Renal clearance of acidic drugs (pKa 3–7) is increased in alkaline urine and decreased in acidic urine. Clinically alkalosis, induced by the administration of sodium bicarbonate infusion, is used for treatment of barbiturate poisoning and acidosis induced by the administration of ammonium chloride or methionine is used for treatment of amphetamine poisoning. 2. The competition for active renal tubular secretion by some drugs will reduce renal clearance, prolong action and cumulating and toxicity of other drugs. Examples are summarised as follows:

Table 3.1 Drugs interacting at renal secretion process

Drug	Renal Secretion or Absorption Competitor	Effect of Interaction
Hydroxyhexamine (active metabolite of acetohexamide)	Phenylbutazone	Hypoglycaemia due to reduced hydroxyhexamine secretion
Indomethacin	Probenecid	Indomethacin secretion reduced
*Penicillin	Probenecid	Penicillin secretion reduced
Sulfinpyrazone	Salicylate	Uricosuria reduced
Pyridostigmine	Ionised tertiary amines	Pyridostigmine secretion reduced
Methotrexate	Probenecid	Methotrexate secretion reduced

*The acidic drug, probenecid, was exploited when penicillin was scarce and costly, it was used to reduce loss of penicillin in the urinary filtrate. Penicillin passes into the urinary filtrate in two ways, $\cong 10\%$ filtration, 90% active tubular secretion. By competitive blocking the active tubular secretion with probenecid, only the relatively small amount of penicillin which filter through the glomerulus is lost in the urine; the probenecid itself being reabsorbed further along the tubule.

PHARMACODYNAMIC DRUG INTERACTIONS

Once a drug reaches the site of action, a second drug may modify the ultimate pharmacological effect by altering the site of drug action in several ways. Understanding these types of interactions usually depends on a thorough knowledge of each biological systems involved and the pharmacological action of drugs. These are predictable.

Competition for The Receptor Sites: Many therapeutic agents may have greater affinity than another drug or endogenous transmitter for a receptor. For example, atropine and d-tubocurarine have little or no intrinsic activity but can occupy a receptor and block the effects of an endogenous active transmitter substance such as acetylcholine (Ach). They produce effects by combining with receptors and thus prevent access of normal physiological transmitter, Ach. The antagonism can be overcome by increasing the amount of agonist at the receptor. Thus, muscle paralysis induced by non-depolarising relaxants such as d-tubocurarine can be reversed by neostigmine that inhibits cholinesterase and increases the concentration of Ach at the receptors. Similarly, competition between isoprenaline and propranolol exists at the β-receptors as the former is an adrenergic agonist the latter an antagonist.

Alteration of the Receptor Sensitivity: Other agents may interact with the active site to modify the intensity of the response through non-competitive processes. For example, in the interaction between *warfarin* and *d-thyroxine*, d-thyroxine, at therapeutic dose, does not alter the ADME of the anticoagulant; and the concentration of the vitamin K-dependent clotting factors is not affected. But d-thyroxine increases the affinity of the warfarin receptor site for warfarin by a factor of 2.4. This increase in receptor affinity for the oral anticoagulant is thought to be responsible for the increased anticoagulant effect in patients treated with both coumarin and indandione anticoagulants. An another example is that of *chlorothiazide* and *digitalis glycosides*, in which chlorothiazide causes hypokalemia thus sensitizes the heart to the biological effects of digitalis. In normal conditions extracellular K^+ competes with digitalis for binding to the enzyme which controls the sodium-potassium pump. During hypokalaemia less K^+ is competing, more digitalis is bound to the enzyme; therefore myocardial contractility increases, resulting arrhythmia.

Drugs acting at the same site on the same physiological system: The depressant effects of hypnotics on the CNS are potentiated by ethanol, narcotic analgesics, antihistamine and tranquillisers. The blood pressure lowering effects of antihypertensive agents is potentiated by diuretics, propranolol, anaesthetics and CNS depressants. These pharmacodynamic actions are not specific.

Alteration of the other Components at the Site of Action: ***Some drugs act by blocking specific metabolising enzymes at the site of action***. For example, the interaction between *neostigmine* and *tubocurarine* during reversal of neuromuscular blockade at skeletal muscle receptors is often used for the reversal after surgery. Neostigmine blocks acetylcholinesterase thus preventing degradation of acetylcholine that displaces tubocuranine from receptors at neuromuscular junction.

Blocking Uptake or Facilitating Release of Noradrenaline, ***5-hydroxytriptamine (5-HT) or other neurotransmitters from storage sites***: For examples, tricyclic antidepressives block the re-uptake of noradrenaline and 5-HT at the synaptic cleft of the nerve endings so that the increased concentrations of these monoamines may modify the post-synaptic receptor numbers or sensitivity for the alleviate depressive disorders. On the other hand MAOIs used for treatment of depression inhibit monoamine oxidase with consequential increase in noradrenaline and 5-HT at the post-synaptic cleft. Guanethidine, bethanidine and debrisoquine are taken up into sympathetic nerve endings by an active transport mechanism that can be blocked competitively by sympathomimetic amines, chlorpromazine, some antihistamine and tricyclic antidepressives. Therefore, prescribing of these two categories of pharmacological agents should be dealt with extreme care.

Great caution is needed when MAOIs are prescribed for patients who are on treatment with other medications such as indirectly acting sympathomimetic agents and amphetamine, tyramine and other sympathomimetic amines. Large amounts of noradrenaline and 5HT are release causing an alarming reaction with severe headache, marked hypertension, acute left ventricular failure, fatal intracerebral haemorrhage. This is the basis of the notorious 'cheese reaction.' Patients should be advised not to take food (cheese and other fermented proteins) containing high contents of amines such as tyramine. Interactions involving MAOI are unpredictable and some occur only in a very small proportion of patients at risk. They are important as the enzyme is irreversibly inhibited, can occur up to 2 to 3 days when after the drugs are discontinued.

Effects on a Different Biological System Which Has Similar or Opposite Effects Thus Augmenting or Diminishing Responses: Sedation may be increased by any combination of alcohol, some antihistamines, barbiturates, narcotic analgesics, phenothiazine neuroleptics; all of which probably have different sites of actions but are all CNS depressants. The interactions between warfarin and aspirin can be interpreted under this category of DI. The small amount of blood loss caused by the direct effect of aspirin on gastric mucosa is usually benign but may be quite hazardous when anticoagulants are administered. Aspirin in large doses, i.e. over 3g per day, may enhance the hypoprothrombinaemic effect of warfarin and possibly other coagulants. When given concurrently in low doses, i.e. under 3g/day aspirin may not affect the anticoagulant effect but inhibit platelet aggregation by interfering with the release of adenosine diphosphate from the platelets and cause undesirable bleeding. Aspirin is 70% protein bound, chronic use of which alters the structure of the serum albumin. It is possible that aspirin may displace warfarin or prevent it from binding with serum albumin. But no evidence indicating this mechanism is clinically important.

REFERENCES

The following list of references is an introduction to the latest available text and journal articles that may help readers to start some interest on the topic. They are selected to give a concise representative picture of clinical and scientific background although there are many other texts in the literature to choose from. The author considers that they are relevant to support the information given in the Chapter.

Gibaldi, M. and Perrier, D. (1992) Drug interactions: Part 1, *Ann. Pharmacother.*, **26**(5), 709–713.
Gibaldi, M. and Perrier, D. (1992) Drug interactions: Part 2, *Ann. Pharmacother.*, **26**(6), 828–834.
Kuhlmann J. (1994) Drug Interaction studies during drug development. In: *Klinische Pharmakologie*, **Vol. 2**, W. Zuckschwerdt Verlag, Munchen, Bern, Wien, New York.
Li, A.P. (1997) *Drug-Drug Interaction: Scientific and regulatory perspectives*, Academic Press, 1997.
Stockley, I.H. (1996) *Drug Interactions: A source book of adverse interactions, their mechanisms, clinical importance and management*. The Pharmaceutical Press, London.

4. CHINESE HERBAL MEDICINE CONCEPTS OF HERBS

KELVIN CHAN

INTRODUCTION

Chinese herbal medicine (CHM), an integral part of the traditional Chinese medicine (TCM), which has several thousand years of history in China, is playing an important role in the medical care of Chinese people even nowadays, in parallel and often integrated with orthodox medical practice. It is the generalisation and summation of the experiences of TCM practitioners' and scholars' long-term struggle against diseases. Its development has evolved into, based on the culture and philosophy of balancing body functions, a medical system through repeated tests and verification in clinical practice. The theories involved may not be easily interpreted in terms of those understood in orthodox medicine.

Through centuries of using various types of CHM materials, possibly initiated by the folklore hero Shen Nong (translated as Divine Plowman) at around 2800 BC, records of cumulative experience were kept. During these early periods, two important works appeared. The Shen Nong Ben Cao Jing (the earlieat recorded materia medica of Shen Nong's herbal experience, translated as The Herbal Classic of the Divine Plowman) recorded 365 herbal materials. The Huang Di Nei Jing (the Inner Canon of the Yellow Emperor, in 100 BC) contained records of diagnosis and treatments using acupuncture and CHM materials. Later, a major updating of herbal experience and medical treatment was carried out by Li Shi Zhen who complied a comprehensive Pharmacopoeia, Ben Cao Gang Mu (Compendium of Materia Medica), in AD 1590, during the Ming Dynasty period. It consisted of 52 volumes, which took the author 30 years for its completion. It lists a total of 1,892 medical substances with more than 1,000 illustrations and about 11,000 prescriptions with detailed description of the appearance, properties, methods of collection, processing procedures and use of each herbal substance. These texts were first translated into Latin and then other languages during the 17th century. In recent years, more herbs have come into use through development, experience and research. There are now about 4,000 herbs, but generally some 500 are in common use. They are grouped under 18 classes according to their effects for treatment.

Chinese herbal medicinal (CHM) substances (often known as Chinese Materia Medica) are made up of plants, animals and minerals with the majority being various parts of medicinal plants. The parts of plants used as crude herbs are processed roots, rhizomes, fruits, seeds, flowers, leaves, woods, barks, vine stems and sometimes, the whole plants. Most of these CHM natural materials are incorporated as composite prescriptions (formulae) that contain 3 to as many as 30 herbs. The herbal mixture is prepared as aqueous decoction by boiling all the herbal ingredients in a fixed amount of water. After simmering down to about one-third of the original volume the warm decoction is consumed orally. Apart from the commonly used decoctions other types of preparations are also administered. These are Powder (*San-ji*), Pill (*Wan-ji*), Extract (*Gao-ji*), Ointment (*Ruan-gao*) Plaster (*Ying-gao*), Liquor (*Jiu-ji,* an alcoholic solution), Medicated tea (*Cha-ji*), and Tablet (*Pian-ji*). Some of the well-known prescriptions have been manufactured into ready-made CHM products in dosage forms, similar to those of orthodox medicinal products that are convenient for patient use. Noticeable problems are those involved with quality control of these products.

CHARACTERISTICS AND FUNCTIONS OF CHINESE MEDICINAL (CM) HERBS

Each Chinese herb has its own specific characters or properties and functions. According to the principles of traditional Chinese medicine, a health body is considered to have a complete balance and harmony between *Yin* and *Yang* aspects of the whole body. Occurrence of disease state is an indication of imbalance of *Yin* and *Yang*. Different characteristics of herbs are employed to treat different kinds of diseases, or to rectify hyperactivity or hypo-activity of *Yin* and *Yang*. Consequently the herbs can cure or prevent the diseases and restore health by restoring the balance of *Yin* and *Yang*. The characters and functions of herbs are classified into 4 groups as follows:

Four Properties (or *Qi*, or energies) of CM Herbs

Each herb has its property or *Qi* (energy) and flavour or taste. Energy refers to the cold, hot, warm or cool nature of the herb. These terms describe the therapeutically significant, energetic characteristics of herbs and their actions. These properties are classified according to the different actions of the herbs on the human body and their therapeutic effects. For example, herbs that cure heat syndrome (*Yang* syndrome) have a cold or cool property, whereas herbs that cure cold syndrome (*Yin* syndrome) has hot or warm property. Herbs of cold and cool natures and herbs of warm and hot nature have opposite properties. A cold-natured herb is different from a cool-natured one only in degree; so is a warm-natured herb different from a hot-natured herb. Most cool or cold natured herbs have the effect of clearing heat, purging fire, removing toxic substances and nourishing *Yin*, and are used to cure heat syndromes. On the contrary, herbs with warm or hot nature usually have the effect of dispersing cold, warming up the interior, supporting *Yang* and treating collapse and are therefore used to treat cold syndromes.

In addition, there is the fifth property, the neutral or mild one. When an herb is neither hot nor cold in nature, it is said to be neutral and can be used for either hot or cold syndromes. Yet, herbs of neutral nature usually tend to be either slightly warm or slightly cool. In general herbs are grouped into four properties only.

Here are two examples to illustrate the nature of herbs. (1) When a person suffers from wind-cold with such symptoms as fever, a version of cold, running nose, clear urine, white tongue coating, he gets a cold syndrome. We use Zi Su Ye (*Folium Perillae*) and Sheng Jiang (*Rhizoma Zingiberis Recens*) to enable the patient to dispel pathogenic factor from the exterior for the body by diaphoresis, thus removing the above symptoms. These two herbs are of hot nature. (2) When a person suffers from carbuncle with such symptoms as pain on the affected part which is red, inflamed and swelling, yellowish urine, yellowish tongue coating, etc. he has a heat syndrome. We use Jin Yin Hua (*Flos Lonicerae*) and Ju Hua (*Flos Chrysanthemi*) to clear away heat and toxic material. These two herbs are of cold nature.

Five Tastes (Flavours) of CM Herbs

The Flavours or Tastes of herbs are often described as pungent (acrid), sweet, sour, bitter, salty, bland (tasteless) and astringent. Since sweet and tasteless are often grouped together and sour and astringent herbs have similar effects, pungent, sweet, sour, bitter and salty are habitually referred as *5 cardinal flavours*. Herbs of different flavours have intrinsic relationship with their efficacy and different compositions show different pharmacological and therapeutic actions. Understanding the characteristics of the 5 tastes is of great importance in guiding the use of herbs for treatment. Herbs of the same taste usually have similarities in effect and even in composition. The flavours do not necessarily refer to the real taste of the drugs. Sometimes they are sorted out according to their true actions rather than tastes. Therefore the flavours of some drugs described in books on materia medica are often different from their true tastes.

Herbs with Pungent (or Acrid) Flavour have the effects of dispersing exo-pathogens from superficies in the body and promoting the circulation of the vital *Qi* (energy) and blood. They are usually used for the treatment of superficial and mild illnesses due to affection by exo-pathogens, stagnation of vital energy, blood stasis, etc. Examples of herbs are Ma Huang (*Herba Ephedrae*) and Chuan Xiong (*Rhizoma Ligustici Chuanxiong*).

Herbs with Sweet Flavour have the effects of nourishing replenishing, tonifying or enriching the different parts or organs of the body, normalising the function of the *Stomach* and *Spleen*, harmonising the properties of other herbs, relieving spasm and pain etc. They are usually effective in treating syndromes of deficiency type, dry cough, constipation due to dry intestine, inco-ordination between the *Spleen* and the *Stomach*, various pains, etc. Some of sweet herbs have detoxification effects. Examples are Huang Qi (*Radix Astragali*) and Gan Cao (*Radix Glycyrrhizae*).

Herbs with Sour Flavour have the effects of inducing astringency and arresting discharge. Sour herbs are often used to treat sweating due to debility, chronic cough, chronic diarrhea, emission, enuresis, frequent micturition, chronic leukorrhagia, etc. Examples are Wu Wei Zi (*Fructus Schisandrae*) and Shan Zhu Yu (*Fructus Corni*).

Herbs with Bitter Flavour have the effects of clearing heat, purging fire, sending down the adverse flow of *Qi* to treat cough and vomiting, relaxing the bowels and eliminating dampness. Such herbs are mostly used for syndromes of pathogenic fire, cough with dyspnea, vomiting, constipation due to heat of excess type, damp-heat syndrome, or cold-damp syndrome. Examples are Huang Lian (*Rhizoma Coptidis*) and Cang Zhu (*Rhizoma Atractylodis*).

Herbs with Salty Flavour have the effects of relieving constipation by purgation, and softening and resolving hard mass. Salty herbs are mostly used in treating dry stool due to constipation, goiter and mass in the abdomen. Examples are Mang Xiao (*Natrii Sulfas*) and Mu Li (*Concha Ostreae*).

Herbs with Tasteless Flavour have the effects of excreting dampness and inducing diuresis and are commonly used for oedema, dysuria, etc. Examples are Yi Ren (*Semen Coicis*) and Hua Shi (*Talcum*).

Herbs with Astringent Flavour have similar actions as those of sour flavour. Examples are Long Gu (*Os Dragonis*) and Wu Mei (*Fructus Mume*).

Herbs of the same flavour generally have similar actions and herbs of different tastes have quite different action. Yet some herbs may have the similar property but different flavour, or similar flavour but different property. Therefore, their effects are not all the same. The property and flavour of herbs should be treated as an integrated whole when they are prescribed.

The Lifting (Ascending), Lowering (Descending), Floating and Sinking Actions of CM Herbs

These actions refer to the upward, downward, outward or inward directions in which CM herbs tend to act on the body. Lifting or ascending (Sheng) means going up or sending up while lowering or descending (Jiang) refers to the opposite. Floating (Fu) means going outward or sending to the surface, whereas sinking (Chen) means going inside or purging into. On the basis of differences in the trends of pathogenesis and affected parts of the body the practitioners make the best use of the directional actions of the herbs to expel and eliminate the pathogenic factors. The herbs may regulate the affected *Qi* flow of the organs and restore the physiological activities to normal. *Lifting and floating herbs* with upward and outward actions are used for elevating *Yang*, relieving exterior syndromes by means of diaphoresis, dispelling superficial wind and cold, inducing vomiting, causing resuscitation. *Lowering* and *sinking* herbs with downward and inward actions are used for clearing heat, purgation, promoting micturition, removing dampness, checking the exuberance of *Yang*, sending down an adverse flow of *Qi* to stop vomiting, relieving cough and asthma, improving digestion to remove stagnated food, tranquillising the mind. The locations of diseases are different in the upper part, in the lower, in the interior and in the exterior of the body. Therefore directions or tendencies of diseases are divided into upward (vomiting) downward (diarrhoea, menorrhagia), outward (spontaneous or night sweating) and inward (internal transmission of exterior syndrome). The lifting, lowering, floating and sinking actions of herbs are used in accordance with the locations of diseases but in opposition to the tendencies of diseases. Generally speaking, in treating diseases located in the upper part or the exterior, it is appropriate to use lifting and floating herbs. In treating diseases located in the lower part of the interior (such as dry stool or constipation) it is proper to use lowering and sinking herbs.

For diseases with manifestations tending upward, herbs of lowering action should be given rather than those with lifting properties. For examples, in the treatment of headache and vertigo due to hyperactivity of the *Liver-yang*, herbs of lowering and sinking actions should be used to calm the *Liver* and suppress hyperactivity of the *Liver-yang*. On the contrary, for diseases with manifestations tending downward, it is suitable to use lifting herbs instead of lowering herbs. For example, in the treatment of chronic diarrhoea due to sinking of *Qi* of the *MiddleJiao*, it is wise to choose lifting herbs to invigorate *Qi* thus lifting *Yang*.

The lifting, lowering, floating and sinking actions of CM herbs have close relationship with their properties and flavours. Most herbs that are pungent or sweet in flavour and warm or hot in property have lifting and floating actions. Most herbs that are bitter, sour or salty in flavour and cold or cool in property have lowering and sinking action. The lifting, lowering floating and sinking actions also have some relationship with the textures of the herbs. Generally speaking, most of the light substances have the action of lifting and floating, but most of the heavy herbs have the action of lowering and sinking. However, though some drugs are light, they have lowering and sinking action; and conversely some heavy drugs have lifting and sinking actions.

These four directional actions of herbs can also be influenced or even altered through the processing and the combine use of herbs. For example, lowering and sinking herbs can have lifting and floating actions after processing with wine, while lifting and floating herbs can have lowering and sinking actions after preparation with salt solution. If lifting and floating herbs are dispensed with a great amount of lowering and sinking ones together, they may also have lowering and sinking actions. Similarly, when lowering and sinking herbs are used together with a great amount of lifting and floating ones, they may exhibit some lifting and floating characteristics.

Classification of CM Herbs According to Channels

This classification refers to the theory of attributive *Channels or Meridians* (*Gui-jing*) of herbs that generalises herb actions in accordance with the theories of *Zang-fu* organs (TCM anatomical organs such as *Heart*, *Liver*, *Spleen*, *Lungs*, *Kidneys*, and other TCM anatomy tissues) and *Channels*. It shows an herb's selective therapeutic effects on a certain part of the *Zang-fu* organs by entering the related *Channel*. An herb may exert obvious or specific therapeutic action on the pathological changes in a certain channel or several channels, but with little effects on the others. For instances, among the heat-clearing herbs, some only clear the heat either in the *Lung Channel* or in the *Liver Channel* or in the *Lung* or in the *Heart Channel*, etc. Among the herbs used as tonics, some strengthen the *Lung* while other strengthen the *Spleen* or the *Kidney*.

Classification of herbs according to Channels is based on the theory of viscera, the theory of Channels and Collaterals, and is summed up according to the curing of particular diseases for which a herb is effective. The human body is an organic whole in which the Channels and Collaterals link up with the interior and exterior and all parts of the body. A pathological change in the exterior may affect the viscera while diseases in the viscera may, in turn find expressions in the exterior of the body. For this reason, the signs and symptoms of diseases occurring in different parts of the body can be understood systematically according to the theory of Channels and Collaterals. For instance, the flaring up of stomach-fire may result in swollen gum, and whenever there is stagnation of *Liver-Qi*, pain in the hypochondriac region will be present. Since the swelling and pain of the gum disappear when Shi Gao (*Gysum Fibrosum*) is administered, and hypochondriac pain relieved with the use of Chai Hu (*Radix Bupleuri*), we may infer that Shi Gao (*Gysum Fibrosum*) acts on disorders of the *Stomach Channel* and Chai Hu (*Radix Bupleuri*) on the *Liver Channel*.

This theory should be associated with the theories of the four properties and five flavours, and actions of lifting lowering, floating and sinking of herbs. Different herbs acting on the same *Channel* have different effect owing to their different properties, flavours, and actions of lifting, lowering, floating and sinking. For example, Huang Qin (*Radix Scutellariae*), Gan Jiang (*Rhizoma Zingiberis*), Bai He (*Bulbus Lilii*) and Ting Li Zi (*Semen Lepidii*) all act on the *Lung Channel*. But Huang Qin can clear lung-heat, Gan Jiang can warm *Lung-cold*, Bai He can be used to make up *Lung-deficiency* and Ting Li Zi is used to soothe excess syndrome of the *Lung*. Therefore only when attention is paid to the different aspects of herbs can their actions be comprehensively analysed and the herbs correctly prescribed. According to the TCM theory, the viscera, *Channels* and *Colleterals* are physiologically related to one another, and pathologically affect one another. When there is pathological change in one *Channel*, herbs acting on other *Channels* should be used in addition to those prescribed for the diseased *Channel* itself.

Classification of CM Herbs According to Toxicity and Non-toxicity

Some CM herbs are toxic in nature. In books on herbal medicine, they are often referred to as slightly toxic, moderately toxic and extremely poisonous. These indicate that the therapeutic dosage of these herbs approaches the toxic dosage, or is already within the toxic dosage, and over dosage may lead to toxic reaction. The herb may give rise to severe side effects within this therapeutic dosage.

For safety use, it is advisable to choose herbs and their proper dosages according to their toxicity, side effects and the patient's constitution such as, age, severity and location of the disease. The dosage of extremely poisonous herbs should be strictly controlled and their over-dosing should be avoided. Such herbs should be discontinued immediately after the patient has got better. Besides, the toxicity of poisonous drugs can be eliminated or lessened by means of processing, dispensing and preparation. Examples of toxic herbs are She Chuang Zi (*Fructus Cnidii*) and Ku Xing Ren (*Semen Armeniacae Amarum*; Slightly toxic), Fu Zi (*Radix Aconiti Lateralis*) and Ban Xia (*Rhizoma Pinelliae*; moderately toxic) and Quan Xie (Scorpio, *Buthus Martensii Karsch*) and Wu Tou (*Radix Aconitum Carmichaeli Debx.*; extremely poisonous).

THE PRESCRIPTIVE USE AND APPLICATION OF CM HERBS

The prescriptive use and application of CM herbs should be made under the direction of the TCM theories and in accordance with the actual disease conditions. Apart from knowing the characters and functions of herbs, the four aspects (**Compatibility, Contraindication, Dosage and Administration**) on the prescriptive use and application of herbs should be observed.

The Compatibility of Herbs (Yao Wu Pei Wu) refers to matching and combination of more than two herbs compatibly and purposely according to specific disease conditions, the requirements of treatment and properties and actions of the chosen herbs. This experience information and knowledge constitutes the foundation to form prescriptions for treatment (Fu Fang Xue). In TCM, disease conditions are considered complex and change-able. Several others may accompany one disease as influenced by changes in the exterior and interior of the body in the form of excess and deficiency in *Yin* or *Yang*, *Cold* or *Heat* in the same case. Thus the use of one herb usually fails to produce the desired therapeutic results. Proper combination of herbs is considered essential to enhance therapeutic effects, cure more related disorders and reduce toxic side effects of some chosen herbs. Ancient TCM practitioners discovered that the combined use of herbs could produce a variety of complicated changes; these were recorded as increase or reduction of herb efficacy. Inhibition or elimination of toxic effects increases in toxicity, and unfavourable adverse reactions. The Shen Nong Ben Cao Jing (Shen Nong's Classic of Herbalism) summarizes these changes into seven categories, which are euphemistically termed as '*Seven Emotions*'.

Single Application (Dan Xing) refers to the use of only one herb to treat the disease.

Synergism or *Mutual Reinforcement* (Xiang Xu) means herbs of similar characters and functions are used in co-ordination to reinforce their effects. For example, the use of both Da Huang (*Radix et Rhizoma Rhei*) and Po Xiao (*Natrii Sulphas*) together increases their purgative effects; Jin Yin Hua (*Flos Lonocerae*) and Lian Qiao (*Fructus Forsythiae*), when used in combination, produce increase in their heat-purging effects.

Mutual Assistance or *Mutual Enhancement* (Xiang Shi) refers to the situation that herbs similar in certain aspects of their characters and functions can be used together, with one as the principal and the others as subsidiary, to help increase the effect of the principal effects. For example, Huang Qi (*Radix Astragali*), which replenishes *Qi* and strengthens the *Spleen* is used together with Fang Ji (*Radix Stephaniae Tetrandrae*), which has diuretic effect, to treat weakness of the *Spleen* accompanied by oedema.

Mutual Inhibition (Xiang Wei) describes the condition when herbs are used in com-bination, the toxicity and side effects of one herb can be reduced or eliminated by the presence of the other. For example, Ban Xia (*Rhizoma Pinelliae*) and Tian Nan Xing (*Rhizoma Arisarmatis*) can inhibit the effects of Sheng Jiang (*Rhizoma Zingiberis Recens*).

Mutual Detoxification (Xiang Sha) implies that one herb can lessen or remove the toxicity and side effects of the other when used in combination. For example, Sheng Jiang (*Rhizoma Zingiberis Recens*) can reduce or eliminate the side effects of Ban Xia (*Rhizoma Pinelliae*) in combination. The folklore antidote decoction for treating poisoning due to Ban Xia (*Rhizoma Pinelliae*) consists of Sheng Jiang (*Rhizoma Zingiberis Recens*), Fang Feng (*Radix Ledebouriellae*), and Gan Cao (*Radix Glycyrrhizae*).

Mutual Antagonism (Xiang Wu) refers to when two herbs are used together, the original efficacy of one herb is reduced or even eliminated by that of the other. For example, the replenishing effects on *Qi* of Ren Shen (*Radix Ginseng*) will be eliminated by Lai Fu Zi (*Semen Raphani*) when they are used in combination.

Incompatibility (Xiang Fan) describes that the use of two herbs together results in toxic or side effects.

In conclusion, when two or more herbs are used in one prescription, they will give rise to interactions and should therefore be chosen carefully according to the conditions of the patient and the characters and functions of herbs. '*Mutual Reinforcement* or *Synergism*' and '*Mutual Assistance* or *Enhancement*' can be employed to improve therapeutic effects by making herbs work in co-ordination and should be used as much as possible. *Mutual*

Detoxification and *Mutual Inhibition* can reduce or eliminate toxicity and side effect of herbs and therefore can be considered when using poisonous herbs for treatment. Herbs with *Mutual Antagonism* and *Incompatibility* will weaken or eliminate efficacy of herbs, or even give rise to toxic and side effects. They should be avoided in combination prescriptions.

Contraindications: Early records in Shen Nong Ben Cao Jing (The Herbal Classic of the Divine Plowman), those reviewed in Ben Cao Gang Mu (Compendium of Materia Medica) and those in recent edition of Chinese Pharmacopoeia (1995) indicate that apart from their effects in preventing or treating disease, some CM herbs can also produce harmful side effects. It is necessary to acquire a clear understanding of these information about them. Examples of these are: Herbs with *Cold* and *Cool* properties can purge *Heat* and may also produce damage to *Yang Qi*. *Hot* herbs can eliminate *Cold*, but may also consume *Yin*. Herbs with powerful purgative actions can eliminate pathogenic factors and impair the antipathogenic *Qi* too. Tonic herbs strengthen the antipathogenic *Qi* yet may also agitate pathogenic *Qi* and making them linger in the body. Herbs with ascending and lifting actions, if used in cases of Yang hyperactivity may worsen the situation. Herbs for suppressing the abnormal ascent of *Qi*, if applied in cases of *Qi* prolapse, may cause the disease case deteriorating further. In order to be sure in administering the right herbs, it is necessary to reduce or moderate the excessive undesirable quality of herbs through processing, seeking proper combinations in making the prescriptions, reducing dosage and improving methods of herbal administration. The harmful effects of CM herbs on the body and precaution in their applications are referred to as 'contraindications'. Historic records of TCM literature list some herbs are incompatible with each other and can never be used in combination; otherwise toxic reactions or weakened therapeutic effects will result. Two groups of 'contraindication' herbs recorded in TCM literature are 'The Eighteen Incompatible Medicaments (*Shi Ba Fan*)' and 'The Nineteen Antagonistic Medicaments (*Shi Jiu Wei*)'. They play a significant role in the choice of composite prescriptions. Apart from historical experience from literature recent experimental studies have shown that some of these potent herbs will produce greater toxicity when given in combination and some do not produce toxicity. So far there is no identical view and further study is needed. It is prudent to use them cautiously and under no circumstances should these herbs be used in combination before sound experimental basis and clinical experience are obtained.

The Eighteen Incompatible Medicaments (Shi Ba Fan) are:

Wu Tou (*Radix Aconiti*) is incompatible with Ban Xia (*Radix Pinelliae*), Gua Lou (*Fructus Trichosanthis*), Bei Mu (*Bulbus Fritillariae Cirrhosae*), Bai Lian (*Radix Ampelopsis*) and Bai Zi (*Rhizoma Bletillae*).

Gan Cao (*Radix Glycyrrhizae*) is incompatible with Da Ji (*Radix Euphorbiae Pekinensis*), Gan Sui (*Radix Kansui*), Yuan Hua (*Flos Genkwa*), and Hai Zao (Seaweed, *Sargassum*).

Li Lu (*Rhizoma et Radix Veratri*) is incompatible with Ren Shen (*Radix Ginseng*), Sha Shen (*Radix Adenophorae*), Dan Shen (*Radix Salviae Miltiorrhizae*), Xuan Shen (*Radix Scrophulariae*), Xi Xin (*Herba Asari*) and Bai Shao (*Radix Paeoniae Lactiflorae*).

The Nineteen Antagonistic Medicaments (Shi Jiu Wei) are:

Liu Huang (*Sulfur*) antagonises Po Xiao (*Mirabilite, Nattrii Sulas*); Sui Yin (*Mercury, Hydrargyrum*) antagonises Pi Shuang (*Arsenic trioxide, Arsenicum*); Lang Du (*Radix Euphorbiae Fischeriae*) antagonises Mi Tuo Seng (*Lithargyrum*); Ba Dou (*Frutus Crotonis*) antagonise Qian Niu Zi (*Semen Pharbitidis*); Ding Xiang (*Clove flower, Flos Caryophylli*) antagonises Yu Jin (*Radix Curcumae*); Chuan Wu (*Radix Aconiti*) and Radix Cao Wu (*Aconiti Kusnezoffii*) antaogonise Xi Jiao (*Cornu Rhinocerotis*); Ya Xiao or Po Xiao (*Mirabilite, Nitrum Depuratum*) antagonises San Leng (*Burreed tuber, Rhizoma Sparganni*); Guan Gui or Rou Gui (*Cortex Cinnamomi*) antagonises Chi Shi Zhi (Red halloysite, *Halloysitum Rubrum*); and Ren Shen (*Radix Ginseng*) antagonises Wu Ling Zhi (*Faeces Trogopterori*).

Contraindications in Use of Herbs during Pregnancy: During pregnancy, improper use of herbs may cause damage to the *Primordial Qi* that is vital for the development of the foetus or else result in abortion as some herbs can harm the original *Qi* of the foetus leading to threatened abortion or miscarriage. TCM practitioners since ancient times have attached great importance to herb contraindications for pregnancy. Most of the prohibited herbs are very poisonous or drastic. Herbs with strong toxicity or purgative effects, and aromatic herbs with motive and dispersive actions should generally be forbidden or only applied with care. These are Ba Dou (*Frutus Crotonis*), Qian Niu Zi (*Semen Pharbitidis*), Da Ji (*Radix Euphorbiae Pekinensis*), Gan Sui (*Radix Kansui*), Yuan Hua (*Flos Genkwa*), and San Leng (*Rhizoma Sparganni*). Herbs that should be given cautiously are usually those that remove blood stasis to restore menstruation, or relieve stagnation by lowering and sinking actions. Examples of these are Tao Ren (*Semen Persicae*), Hong Hua (*Flos Carthami*), Da Huang (*Radix et Rhizoma Rhei*), Fu Zi (*Radix Aconiti Lateralis Preparata*), and Rou Gui (*Cortex Cinnamomi*). Unless it is absolutely necessary, poisonous and drastic herbs should not be used during pregnancy. For a pregnant woman with serious illness that cannot be treated without one or more of these herbs they can be prescribed with great care according to the patient's disease conditions.

Dosage: In the TCM concepts of treating diseases with herbs, attention should be paid to the dosage as it has a direct influence on the therapeutic effects. Too small a dosage for a serious case would fail to obtain the desired results, but too large a dosage for a mild case would usually cause damage to the antipathogenic *Qi* resulting wastage of the medicinal herbs. Usually, the dosage of using herbs is calculated by weight, though a few case are based on quantity or volume. Throughout the development of the Chinese history a traditional weight system had been developed to deal with daily life activities. One *Jin* equals to 16 *Liang* and one *Liang* equals ten *Qian*. The recently developed metric system has now been adopted. An appropriate value to equate the two systems has been adopted to interpret the ancient TCM weights for prescribing CM herbs in metric system: 1Liang = 30 grammes; 1Qian = 3grammes; 1Fen = 0.3gramme; and 1Li = 0.03gramme.

Dosage quoted in most TCM literature refers to the daily amount of each herb for an adult, and also the relative amount of different herbs in a recipe or prescription. Since most of the CM herbs are crude herbs, the range of safe dosage is usually wide and the therapeutic range is not as narrow and restricted as that for orthodox synthetic drugs. Some of the herbs are, however, very drastic and potent in nature or containing extremely poisonous chemicals. The dosage of each of these poisonous or potent herbs should be strictly controlled to prevent poisoning. Understanding all the factors that would affect the choice of dosage of CM herbs is of paramount importance. These are:

The Relationship between Characteristics of Herbs and Dosage: For herbs with mild properties, the dosage can be large; for toxic or potent herbs it should be small. For herbs of light-weight, the dose used should be small and that for non-toxic herbs should be large. For effective but very expensive herbs such as Ren Shen (*Radix Ginseng*), Niu Huang (*Calculus Bovis*), etc., the dosage should be small so as not to cause wastage. In very seldom circumstance of using fresh medicinal herbs that contain some water, the dosage should be approximately twice the dried ones.

The Relationship between the Dosage and Dosage Forms of the Prescriptions: Generally speaking, the dosage of a prescription containing only one herb should be larger than that of a compound prescription that contains multiple herbs. And when the prescription of herbs is used in decoction, the dosage should be larger than that is used in bolus and powder form. For example, if Rou Gui (*Cortex Cinnamoni*) is prescribed for use in a decoction the usual dosage is 3g, but for use as a powder, the dosage is 0.5 to 1.5g. Dosage of the principal herbs in a prescription should be larger than those of the adjuvant or subsidiary herbs.

The Relationship between Dosage and the Disease Conditions, Constitution and Age of the Patient: Usually the dosage for serious conditions, emergencies and stubborn problems should be larger, while for mild and chronic conditions, smaller. The dosage can be large for the strong patient and smaller for the aged, the frail, the maternal and children. As a rule, the dosage for a child over six years old is half the dosage for an adult. The dosage for one under five is a quarter, and for an infant, even smaller. In addition, attention should be paid to the dosage of the toxic herbs.

In summary, when prescribing CM herbs for treatment, three major aspects should be taken into account in deciding the dosage of herbs. They are intrinsic properties of the herbs, rational composition of the prescriptions and patients' disease conditions. The dosage and prescription composition should be adjusted according to variations in individual constitution, geographical location and climatic and seasonal influences.

Dietetic Restraint: In the course of treatment with herbs, foods unfit for the disease or contraindicated to certain herbs should be restrained. Indigestible and irritating food should be restrained or avoided. For instance, for *cold* syndromes, uncooked or cold food should be avoided; for *heat* syndromes, hot, pungent, and greasy food is not advisable. Patients with dizziness, insomnia and impetuous temperament should not take food with pepper, wine, garlic, etc. Patients with indigestion due to deficiency of the *Spleen* and *Stomach*, fried, greasy and sticky food should be avoided. Patients with infection on body surface and cutaneous pruritus, should not take fish, shrimps, crabs, and other fishy and irritating food. Some CM herbs are often used as dietary supplement depending on the amount and frequency of use. Patients are often prescribed tonic herbs for their chronic illnesses. Knowledge of the patients' eating habit is essential for successful prescription.

Administration: CM herbs can be taken internally and applied externally. External preparations include moxa-application, medicinal decoction for bathing, throat insufflation, eye-drops, dressings or plasters with medicinal powder, liquor (an alcoholic extract of herbs) for external use, ointment, suppository, etc. The type of preparations used depends on disease conditions and characteristics of chosen herbs. In treating rheumatic pain and traumatic injuries, medicinal liquors should be recommended so that their ability to activate blood circulation and remove stagnation from the meridian can be achieved readily. The active ingredients of some herbs such as *Radix Kansui* and *Gemma Agrimoniae*, are not soluble in water, the extract herbs should be processed into pills or powder. Internal preparations include oral decoction, oral infusion, liquor extract, powder, pill, medicated tea, medicinal granules, capsule and tablet. Injections of herbal extracts for infusion are available for parenteral administration.

In TCM, medicinal decoction is a very common form of Chinese pharmaceutical preparation for oral administration. Therefore, the methods of preparing decoction should be observed, followed and administered.

Methods for Preparing A Decoction: A ceramic pot (or other earthenware of enamel or glass material) is preferred to any metal pot to decoct herbs in order to prevent likely reactions with the vessel material. The herbs should be soaked in clean drinking water for 30 minutes before they are decocted. The amount (250 to 300ml) used should be just enough to submerge the herbs. In general, one dose (one packet of herbal mixture) is decocted twice and the resulting two decoctions are taken orally on separate occasion. Tonic herbs can be decocted thrice. The resulting dark decoction (usually about one-third of the original volume added) after boiling and simmering can be consumed. The temperature during heating with water should be controlled according to the properties of the herbs. Aromatic herbs should be decocted over a strong fire and done quickly in a short period (3 to 5 minutes) to avoid evaporation and reduction of volatile contents. Tonic herbs with dense texture should be decocted over a gentle flame for a longer period (40 to 60 minutes) to obtain the effective ingredients into the simmering water. Different herbs in the same prescription need different decocting methods to guarantee the quality of the decoction and keep the therapeutic effects of the herbs. Clear instructions must be written in the prescription so that the TCM pharmacist or the patient can follow to prepare the decoction properly. These instructions are:

To be Decocted First (Xian Jian): This step is essential for some mineral or shell herbs as they are hard in texture and their active components cannot be extracted easily. They, crushed in small pieces, should be boiled for 10 to 15 minutes before others are put in the pot. Examples are Gao Shi (*Gypsum Fibrosum*) and Mu Li (*Concha Ostreae*). Toxic herbs, such as Fu Zi (*Radix Aconiti Lateralis Preparata*) and Chuan Wu (*Radix Aconiti*), should be decocted first to reduce or remove their toxicity by boiling prior to addition of other herbs into the decoction.

To be Decocted Later (Hou Xia): Some aromatic herbs should be put in after the others are boiled for a period when almost done. They should be boiled for about 5 minutes in order to prevent the loss of their volatile active components. These herbs include Bo He (*Herba Menthae*), Sha Ren (*Fructus Amomi*). Some purgative herbs such as Da Huang (*Radix et Rhizoma Rhei*) and Fan Xie Ye (*Folium Senna*) should also be boiled later.

To be Decocted with Wrappings (Bao Jian): Some powder-like and sticky herbs that easily make the decoction turbid and unpleasant to taste. Some floats on top of the boiling decoction. Some are with fur or fine hair that irritate the throat. They should be wrapped in a piece of gauze for decoction, so that the decoction will not be turbid, irritating to the throat, or burnt at the bottom of the pot. Examples are Che Qian Zi (*Semen Plantaginis*), Xuan Fu Hua (*Flos Inulae*), and Talcum (ground in water).

To be Decocted Separately (Ling Jian): Some precious herbs such as Ren Shen (*Radix Ginseng*), Xi Yang Shen (*Radix Panacis Quiquefolii*) should be decocted separately. The decoction obtained can be mixed with the finished decoction of other herbs to avoid any waste of active ingredients these precious herbs that may be absorbed by other herbs in the decoction during boiling.

To be Taken with the Decoction: Herbs unsuitable for decoction should be ground into fine powder and infused with warm boiled water or finished decoction. Examples are San Qi (*Radix Notoginseng*), liquid herb such as Sheng Jiang, ginger juice, (*Rhizoma Zingiberis Recens*) should be taken following its infusion as well.

To be Melted in Boiled Solution (*Yang Hua*): Some of the gluey and very sticky herbs should be melted or dissolved in boiling water or finished decoction for oral administration. For examples are E Jiao (*Colla Corii Asini*), Yi Tang etc.

Instructions for Use of CM Preparations: In general, one dose (two decoctions of the same recipe) should be taken twice a day. For acute, emergency or severe cases, two doses (four decoctions) or more may be given per day at an interval of four hours. During the treatment of chronic illnesses one dose can be taken for two days (one decoction per day). Herbal decoctions for stopping vomiting can be repeated in small doses. For unconscious patients and those with lockjaw the decoction can be applied via nasal feeding. Purgative and diaphoretic herbal preparations should be stopped once the patients begin to sweat or have bowel movements; this is to stop excessive sweating or purgation that may damage the antipathogenic *Qi*. Powdered herbal preparations should be taken with boiled warm water. Preparations prescribed in large doses with strong unpleasant smell and taste can be taken together with honey in the decoction.

Concerning the timing of administration, usually tonic preparations should be taken before meals whereas those irritating to the stomach and intestines should be taken after meals (1 to 2 hours before or after meals). Anthelmintics and purgatives should be taken on an empty stomach. Preparations with sedative and tranquilizing effects should be taken one to two hour before bed-time. Medicine for chronic illnesses should be taken at regular time while medicine for acute diseases should be given instantly without a limitation of time.

Herbal decoction is usually taken while it is warm. For patients with vomiting feeling, the decoction can be concentrated and given frequently in small amount. Pill or bolus and powder should be taken with warm boiled water.

THE PROCESSING OF HERBS

Herb processing (Pao Zhi) is the process of treating natural herbs in accordance with the therapeutic, dispensing and pharmaceutical requirements before they are used or further made into various preparations. The processing consisting of primary treatment and subsequent special preparation of natural herbal materials (materia medica). Most TCM materia medica come from natural sources often mixed with impurities and dirts after collection. Some cannot be stored for a long time owing to their tendency to deteriorate. Some cannot be directly used because of their toxicity or drastic actions. Some require special treatment to meet the therapeutic requirements. Special processing refers to a kind of high temperature stir-baking processes. All TCM materia medica must be processed prior to application or preparation into various forms in order to safeguard therapeutic effects and safety of administration.

The Aim of Processing:

(1) To eliminate or reduce the toxicity, drastic actions, and side effects of some herbs. For instance, Ba Dou (*Fructus Crotonis*) is processed into powder and defatted to reduce the toxins that cause strong purgative action. Stir-baking of raw Olibanum and Myrrha that cause nausea and vomiting reduces the undesirable reactions. The toxicity of Wu Tou (*Radix Aconiti*), Tian Nan Xing (*Rhizoma Pinelliae Pedatisctae*) can be lessened through processing by boiling in water.
(2) To enhance or increase the efficacy of herbs. When Zi Wan (*Radix asteris*), Kuan Dong Hua (*Flos Farfarae*) are stir-baked with honey, they have a greater effect of nourishing the lung to arrest cough. Yan Hu Suo (*Rhizoma Corydalis*) processed with vinegar has greater analgesic effects.
(3) To change the character and function of herbs in order to meet the therapeutic needs. For example, Sheng Di Huang (raw *Radix Rehmanniae*) is *Cold* in property and is used to clear *Heat* form the blood. After it is processed by steaming it becomes Shu DI Huang (*Radix Rehmanniae Preparata*), and is *Warm* in property and is mainly used for enriching the blood.
(4) To facilitate decoction, preparation and preservation. When herbal materials are sliced or broken up into smaller pieces, they can be decocted more conveniently. It is easier to extract their active principles, or easier to grind and make them into different forms of medicine. Mineral or shell herbs are easier to be crushed or broken into pieces after calcining and tempering in vinegar.
(5) To get rid of impurities, non-medicinal parts and various bad tastes in order to ensure clean herbs for administration.
(6) To secure preservation and prevent decaying of herbs using adequately drying process.

Methods of Processing:

(1) Primary Processing consists of
   • Cleaning (To get rid of the impurities, earth and sand and non-medicinal parts in the herbs),
   • Crushing or grinding (To crush herbs or break them into pieces or grind them into powder in order to facilitate further preparation and utilization),
   • Cutting or slicing.(To cut herbs according to different requirements, into slices, segments, lumps or fibers to make herbs convenient for decoction and further processing and also make herbs easier to be dried, preserved and prepared into various forms of medicine),
   • Washing (To wash off the earth, sand and impurities on the surface of herbs, to pan impurities with water),
   • Moistening (To sprinkle clean water on herbs repeatedly and then covering them with wet covering to soften them for easy cutting),
   • Rinsing (To put herbs in running water in order to rinse off their salty, stinking or fishy smells), refining powder with water (Shui Fei, To grind insoluble minerals with water into fine powder).

(2) Stir-baking (Chao): refers to baking the crude herbs in a pan with constant stirring. This process for different herbs may vary according to time and temperature and the required appearance of the processed herbs (baked till yellow, brown or carbonised). For example, Bai Zhu (*Rhizoma Atractylodis Macrocephalae*) is baked to yellow in order to obtain the effect to strengthen the *Spleen Qi*; Di Yu (*Radix Sanguisorbae*) is baked to carbonise fragments for improved haemostatic effects.

(3) Stir-baking with adjuvants (Zhi): refers to baking the herbs with liquid adjuvants such as honey, ginger juice, salt water, vinegar, and wine. These liquids, possessing their own therapeutic effects, after processing with the herbs will enhance the herbs' therapeutic effects. For example, Flos Farfarae (Kuan Dong Hua) stir-baked with honey produces an enhanced effect in moistening the lung and relieving cough. Radix Astragali seu Hedysari (Huang Qi) stir-baked with honey produce an improved effect in strengthening the *Middle Jiao* and replenishing *Qi*. Sand stir-baking is also used. The sand is stir-baked in a pan until it is hot and the herbs are mixed with the heated sand to produce herbs that are light and crispy. This process ia often used for crustaceous herbs with hard shells.

(4) High-temperature Stir-baking (Pao): is basically the same procedure as those mentioned above. It is done quickly over high heat to loosen and crack the herbs.For example, Rhizoma Zingiberis is processed to produce Rhizoma Zingiberis Preparata to reduce its pungent and dispersive properties for warming the *Middle Jiao*. Radix Aconiti Lateralis Preparata (Fu Zi) and Semen Strychni (Ma Qian Zi) are heated in a hot charcoal ashes until brown and cracking but not yet carbonised. Such process help to eliminate poisonous ingredients in the raw herbs.

(5) Calcining (Duan): refers to burning a herb directly or indirectly over a fire to make the herb light, crispy, and easily crushable in order to bring out its therapeutic effects. Herbs from mineral or shellfish sources such as *Magetitum* and *Concha Ostreae*, are calcined directly until they turn red. During indirect calcining the herbs, such as *Vagina Trachycaroi Carbonisatus* and *Crinis Carbonisatus* are burned in an air-tight refractory vessel.

(6) Wet-coated baking or roasting (Wei): refers to baking or roasting the herbs coated with wet paper or wet dough in an oven until the coats turn black. This process reduces the fat and moderates the action of some herbs such as Shu Jiang (*Rhizoma Zingiberis Recens Preparata*) and Rou Dou Kou (*Semen Mystristicae Preparata*).

(7) Steaming (Zheng): refers to steaming the herbs together with other adjuvants over a slow fire until they are cooked. For example, Sheng Di (Raw *Radix Rehmanniae*) has a *Cold* nature acting to purge *Heat*. After steaming with wine, it becomes Shu Di (*Radix Rehmanniae Preparata*) that has a *Warm* nature and is effective in replenishing *Yin* and blood. Sheng Da Huang (Raw *Radix et Rhizoma Rhei*), processed by steaming with rice wine, has a reduced purgative effect and is more effective in activating blood circulation and removing blood stagnation as Shu Da Huang (*Radix et Rhizoma Rhei Preparata*).

(8) Boiling (Zhu): refers to boiling the herbs in water together with adjuvant. Chuan Wu (*Radix Aconiti*), boiled with beancurd, and Yuan Hua (*Flos Gankwa*), boiled in vinegar become less toxic as the processing removes the toxic chemicals.

(9) Other methods are: Herbs can be processed in some special ways as required, such as germination, fermentation, and frostation. Germination means to let seeds sprout to a proper length and dry them for use. Fermentation means that an herb is allowed to ferment at a certain temperature. Frostation is the process of defatting seed herbs partially. For example, Mang Xiao (*Mirabilite*) is put into watermelon and left in a well-ventilated place until frost-like powder emerges on its surface.

REFERENCES

The following list of references consists of books and papers written in English. These are considered as introductory text for readers who may begin to get interested in traditional Chinese medicine (TCM). TCM students can use them as textbooks or reference books for their courses in Chinese materia medica. The author has managed to obtain information on the text in English and compare with the Chinese text available from his travels to the major TCM universities in China. Some of the text available in English outside of the TCM universities in China may not have the 'philosophical realness' or factual correctness compared with the very abundant Chinese texts used by the students in these universities. English speaking students who wish to get a real grip or master the understanding of TCM should attempt to learn the Chinese text if at all possible. Nevertheless the chosen few books here should be helpful as a start.

Kaptchuk, T.J. (1983) *The Web That Has No Weaver: Understanding Chinese Medicine*, Congdon & Weed, Inc., Chicago. ISBN: 0-8092-2933-1Z

Geng, J-Y. and Su Z-h. (1990) *Practical Chinese Medicine & Pharmacology: Basic Theories and Principles*, New World Press, Beijing. ISBN: 7-80005-113-7

Geng, J-Y., Huang, W-Q., Ren, T-C. and Ma, X-f. (1991) *Practical Traditional Chinese Medicine & Pharmacology: Medicinal Herbs*, New World Press, Beijing. ISBN: 7-80005-119-6.

Geng, J-Y., Huang, W-Q., Ren, T-C. and Ma, X-f. (1991)) *Practical Traditional Chinese Medicine & Pharmacology: Herbal Formulas*, New World Press, Beijing. ISBN: 7-80005-117-X

State Administration of Traditional Chinese Medicine, (1995) *Advanced Textbook on Traditional Chinese Medicine: Book 1: Traditional Chinese Pharmacy*, New World Press, Beijing. ISBN: 7-80005-262-1

State Administration of Traditional Chinese Medicine, (1995) *Advanced Textbook on Traditional Chinese Medicine: Book 2: Science of Traditional Chinese Prescription*, New World Press, Beijing. ISBN: 7-80005-262-2

Xu G-J. and Chan, K. (1994) *Pictorial Compendium of Poisonous Traditional Chinese Herbs Available in Hong Kong (First Edition In Chinese)*. Commercial Press, Hong Kong. ISBN: 962-07-3136-0

Chan, K. (1995) *Progress in traditional Chinese medicine. Trends in Pharmacological Sciences*, **16**, 182–187.

Chan, K. (2000) *Pictorial Compendium Of Poisonous Traditional Chinese Medicinal Natural Products* (In English), Harwood, Amsterdam, in press.

5. CHINESE HERBAL MEDICINE CONCEPTS OF PRESCRIPTIONS

KELVIN CHAN

HISTORICAL DEVELOPMENT OF TCM PRESCRIPTIONS

A prescription used for treatment in traditional Chinese medicine (TCM) can be defined as a recipe or formula of herbs that, after correct diagnosis based on the differentiation of syndromes and establishment of therapeutic methods, combines appropriate herbs for the prevention and treatment of diseases. The scientific study of principles of formulating prescriptions is Fu Fang Xue that is the foundation for the science of TCM prescriptions.

The formation and development from using single herbs to multiple-herbs prescriptions in China have undergone a very long historical period. In the Shang Dynasty (1600 B.C), because of the increased variety of herbs and the enrichment of knowledge about diseases, more herbs were selected according to the different symptoms of illnesses to formulate compound prescriptions for clinical use. During the 'Spring & Autumn and the Warring States' period (770-221 BC), a classical writing of TCM dedicated to the Emperor, entitled *"The Inner Canon of the Yellow Emperor"* (*Huang Di Nei Jing*), appeared. This is the earliest book dealing with the basic theories of the science of TCM formulae apart from other recorded medical information. It gives summaries of the theories and principles for syndrome differentiation, treatment, prescription, and herbs used in treating diseases The book consisting of 13 prescriptions has laid down from usage experience the development of TCM formulae. In the Eastern Han Dynasty (25-220 AD), Zhang Zhong-jing, an outstanding physician, compiled a very famous book entitled *"Treatise on Cold Diseases and Miscellaneous Diseases"* (*Shang Han Lun*), which contains 269 prescriptions. All the later physicians have honoured this book as the "Forerunner of all Prescription Books" in TCM. It brings together syndrome differentiation, treatment, prescription, and herbs for treatment and interpretation in detail to the modification of the prescriptions and their administrations. The book gives the foundation for the formation and development of the science of TCM prescription.

Through subsequent dynastic periods, various emperors with the help of medical and pharmaceutical scholars commissioned a great number of prescription books and pharmacopoeia. Many ancient prescriptions, secret prescriptions, and proven prescriptions were collected, researched, systemised and widely applied. Notable publications produced are listed as follows:

Tang Ben Cao (Tang Xin-Xiu Ben Cao, 659 AD, the Tang's Newly Revised Materia Medica), commissioned by the Emperor in Tang Dynasty and written by Su Jing with 23 other medical and pharmaceutical scholars. This publication provides rectified information consequential of mistakes from previous medical texts, and is considered to be the earliest official pharmacopoeia in the world. It contains 54 chapters and 850 herbal descriptions, which included 20 imported herbs from foreign countries. It had great influence on medical practice in China, Japan and Korea and had been used as mandatory text in traditional medical schools during the periods. Internationally, this text was considered as the earliest known official pharmacopoeia published in the world, being over 800 years and 1100 years earlier than the Italian Florence Pharmacopoeia (1499 AD) and the Denmark Pharmacopoeia (1772 AD) respectively.

Tai Ping Hui Min He Ji Ju Fang (An official formulary published in about 1151 AD by the Official Formulary Pharmacy Bureau of the Song Dynasty) was commissioned by the Song Imperial Government. It included 788 types of recipes and formularies with details of stated ingredients, dosage, indications, and processing preparation methods. This work probably unified the recipes and formulations of this time and became the first official quality standard of herbal preparations in history as it protected people from adulterated and misbranded herbal products that had been illegally manufactured.

During the last stage of the Qing Dynasty in China, the corruption and incompetence of the government exposed China to foreign invasion. In medical and social aspects, China suffered the problem of nearly nation-wide of opium addiction that weakened her economical, political and physical power. Under the influence of Westernisation the practice of orthodox medicine became more popular besides other social or political aspects.

The Post-Revolution Period (1911–1960s) marked a significant change in the history of China not only politically but also in medical practice. The Republic of China was born after the 1911 Revolution that was led by an orthodox medical practitioner, Dr. Sun Yat-Sen. During such a turbulence period it was not surprising that hardly any medical progress was made. Croizer pointed out in a review that the record of Chinese medical developments prior to 1949 was not impressive and before 1927 was dismal. Civil wars broke out in China one after the other. No efficient measures were taken to get rid of opium smoking. Under the then Nationalist (Guo-Min Dong) government there were over 20 million opium users in China. The practice of orthodox medicine took over the health care and TCM practice was not allowed or curtailed. Most chemical drugs were supplied by foreign drug companies and no regulations on drug use and drug quality control were available to check on adulterated drugs and misbranded preparations, manufactured domestically or imported, which flooded the market.

Since the founding of the People's Republic of China (PRC) in 1949, in the development of medical practice the government took effective and decisive measures to eradicate opium smoking in just three years. The PRC government re-emphasised the importance of TCM practice by restoring TCM with the intention of breaking the China's dependence on the West. Over 10 TCM colleges and institutes were established in the coastal provinces and in Si-Chuan Province. Orthodox physicians were re-educated with TCM principles and practice. This marked the start of an integration of education and practice of both orthodox medicine and traditional Chinese medicine. Not only the science of TCM prescriptions has been studied, but also the therapeutic mechanism of ancient prescriptions has been researched. A series of textbooks and monographs have been compiled and published, laying down a foundation and reference for further development.

After the Cultural Revolution (1966 to 1976) China was restored to 'normal'. Within a period of 3 to 5 years the Ministry of Public Health was authorised to revise and promulgate up to 24 Regulations and Acts for all use of medicinal products and related businesses. They are concerned with drug administration enforcement, new drug applications, special control of narcotics, psychological drugs, poisons, pharmaceuticals, hospital pharmacy, criteria for punishing violators of drug regulations, drug importation and exportation, introduction of clinical trials, and new drug applications by foreign companies and those through joint ventures between China and foreign companies. Based on these various regulatory development and implementation the first official Chinese Drug Control Law was adopted in 1984. It is believed that continuing development and progress are being made and adopted to comparable international standard.

Meanwhile, a lot of new effective prescriptions have been created and recorded in the literature. Nowadays approved composite formulae of famous prescriptions have been included in the Chinese Pharmacopoeia (English Edition 1992 one volume; Chinese Edition 1995 two volumes) Generally, prescriptions are nowadays classified into 17 kinds according to their effectiveness on different types of diseases.

COMPOSITION OF A TCM PRESCRIPTION

During the development of prescriptions, an early TCM prescription contained only one herb or might be two or more. Some prescriptions gradually became established for specific diseases that were later modified in clinical practice according to differentiation of syndromes. Different herbs have different properties, flavours and tastes, and each has its own specific functions and deficiencies. Thus the purposes of having a combination of herbs in a prescription are (1) To select herbs according to the differentiation of syndromes of the whole diseased body for curing complicated cases; (2) To enhance the therapeutic effects of individual herbs by promoting their synergism; and (3) To inhibit the adverse effects of other potent herbs or to counteract the toxicity of poisonous ones in the prescriptions. In the selection of proper herbs for a prescription, it is necessary to distinguish between the principal herbs and the secondary ones, making sure that they complement and antagonise in the right ways of one another in order to produce the most effective results in the treatment of diseases. The principles for the composition of prescriptions, as first described in the Huang Di Nei Jing (The Inner Canon of the Yellow Emperor), stipulate that a prescription should include four different herbs. They are the Chief or Principal (Jun), the Adjuvant (Chen), the Assistant (Zuo) and the Guide (Shi) according to the different roles they play in the prescription.

The Chief Herb or Principal Herb (Jun), being essential in a prescription, aims to produce the leading effect in treating the cause of the main symptom of a disease. It plays the principal curative role.

The Adjuvant Herb (Chen) helps to strengthen the curative actions of the Chief Herb or treat less important symptoms by its own.

The Assistant Herb (Zuo) aims at producing the leading effect in treating the accompanying diseases or symptoms, helps to strengthen the effect of the principal herb by playing a significant role in treatment, and counteracts the potent effects or toxicity of the Chief and Adjuvant Herbs.

The Guiding Herb (Shi) leads the effects of other herbs to the diseased parts of the body and to balance the actions of the other herbs in the prescriptions.

As a rule, the Chief Herb should be used as the dominating one in a prescription, with the Adjuvant, Assistant and the Guiding Herbs subordinate to it. The four herbs supplementing one another play the curative role together. However, not every prescription is composed of the four kinds of herbs together. It may be composed of the principal herb with any one of the other three kinds depending on the conditions of the diseases, characteristics of the herbs and therapeutic needs. In some prescriptions the Chief Herb or the Adjuvant Herb itself possesses the action of the Assistant or Guide Herb.

MODIFICATION OF A PRESCRIPTION

When composing a prescription, apart from following the above-mentioned principles, one should consider the patient's disease state, the constitution, age and sex of the patient as well as the environment of the patient's dwelling and seasonal changes. It is therefore necessary to modify a set prescription to cope with various situations during the course of treatment of the disease in the following ways:

Modification of Number of Herbs: It is possible to increase or decrease the number of herbs in an established prescription to produce a new prescription with changes in the compatibility of the herbs and in therapeutic effects. For example, Decoction of Ephedrae (consisting of 4 herbs, Ma Huang (*Herbra Ephedrae*), Rou Gui (*Ramulus Cinnamomi*), Ku Xing Ren (*Semen Armeniacae Armarum*), and Gan Cao (*Radix Gltcyrrhizae Preparata*) treats exterior-excess syndromes caused by exposure to *Cold*. Its chief action is to induce perspiration and expel the *pathogenic factor* via the exterior. By removing Rou Gui (*Ramulus Cinnamomi*), the new 'Three Crude Herbs Decoction' is used to release the inhibited *Qi* and expel *Cold*, in illnesses due to exposure to *Wind-Cold* characterised by dysfunction of *Lung Qi*, with symptoms of stuffy nose, hoarse voice, productive cough, full sensation in the chest, shortness of breath, white tongue coating and superficial pulse. Another example of removing Gui Zhi (*Ramulus Cinnamomi*) and adding 4 more herbs to the Decoction of Ephedrae is the Huagui Powder. The 4 addition herbs are Zi Su Zi (*Fructus Perillae*), Chen Pi (*Pericarpium Citri Reticulatae*), Red Fu Ling (*Poria Rubra*) and Shu Bai Pi (*Cortex Mori Radicis Preparata*). This prescription based on Decoction of Ephedrae can release the inhibited *Lung Qi*, and expel *Cold* as well as regulate the *Flow of Qi* and resolve phlegm due to additional symptoms such as asthma, difficult expectoration, and serious full sensation of the chest.

Modification of the Quantity of the Herbal Ingredients: It is possible to alter the compatibility between herbal ingredients of an established prescription by changing their quantities, thus changing its action, potency and indications and extending the scope of the treatment. Decoction for Treating Yang Exhaustion that contains the following 3 herbs: Fu Zi (*Radix Aconiti Lateralis*), Shang Jiang (*Rhizoma Zingiberis*), and Gan Cao (*Radix Glycyrrhizae Preparata*) in the quantities of 1 piece, 1.5 liang and 2 liang respectively. This prescription has the actions of recuperating the depleted *Yang* and rescuing the patient from danger in treating cold limbs due to dominant *Yin* and deficient *Yang*, watery diarrhoea with undigested food, and deep and fine pulse. When changing to the quantities of 1 large piece, 3 liang and 2 liang respectively of the same herbs, 'Decoction of Dredging Meridian for Cold Extremities' can recuperate the depleted *Yang* and activate pulse beat. These actions are useful to treat syndromes such as cold limbs due to dominant *Yin* repelling *Yang*, flushed complexion, watery diarrhoea with undigested food and fading pulse.

Modification of Dosage Forms for the Same Prescription

A prescription can be prepared into various dosage forms, each having its own characteristics. The most suitable and effective dosage form should be selected to meet the need of the patient's illness and convenience for administration for the curative effect. By preparing the herbal ingredients of a prescription into different dosage forms the same prescription may produce different effects for treating different diseases. For example, 'Pill for Regulating the *Middle Jiao*' is used to treat deficiency *Cold* in the *Spleen* and *Stomach* composed of equal amounts of Sheng Jiang (*Rhizoma Zingiberis*), Ren Shen (*Radix Ginseng*), Bai Zhu (*Rhizome Atractyodis Macroephalae*) and Gan Cao (*Radix Glycyrrhizae Preparata*). When the same ingredients are prepared as a decoction it is more potent and produces a faster action and is suitable for an acute or a serious case. Ingredients in the decoction are more readily absorbed after orally administration than the pill that may have a more prolonged action.

The common dosage forms used in TCM prescriptions are as follows:

Decoction (Tang Ji), most commonly used as a medicinal solution, is obtained by boiling for some time the selected herbs in water. It can be absorbed via the oral route easily, producing a speedy and drastic effect. It is used for serious and acute cases.

Pill and Bolus (Wan Ji) are round medicinal mass of various sizes prepared by grinding herbs into powder, mixing with excipients such as honey, water, rice paste, flour paste, wine or vinegar. They are convenient to use and storage, with slow absorption, lasting effects and small dosage. They are normally used for mild and chronic illness. There are four kinds of commonly used pills: honeyed pill, watered pill, pasted pill and condensed pill according to the binding agents or methods that are used for preparation. Examples are: Pill of Six Magic Actions (Liu Shen Wan) for sore throat, Pill for *Yin*-Replenishing.

Medicated Wine or Liquor (Jiu Ji) is a transparent alcoholic solution obtained by soaking or simmering the herbs in white or yellow wine for a certain period of time. The liquor may be taken orally or applied externally. Some medicated wines with the right herbs are used for the treatment of general asthenia, rheumatic pain contusion and strains. Some are often used as a tonic for improving the health e.g. Tonic Wine of Ten herbs

Medicated Tea (Cha Ji) is prepared by mixing pulverised herbs with binder or sticker to form granules or cakes. They are used as drinks by adding boiling water. This preparation is often used for common cold and indigestion. Wushi tea is an example.

Extract (Gao Ji) is prepared by boiling the herbs repeatedly three times and discarding the dregs. The resulting bulked solution is further condensed before sugar or honey is added to form a semi-liquid preparation. It serves as an oral tonic suitable for chronic and debilitating illnesses. For example, Extract of Ginseng & Astragali (Ren Shen and Huang Qi), is a common tonic.

Dan (Dan Ji) is a general term for some preparation made of refined or precious herbs. Dan for oral use is prepared as fine powder or pellets. Dan is used instead of powder as an indication that the herbal ingredients are rare and precious.

Distillate (Yao Lu) is obtained by distilling fresh herbs containing volatile substances. It tastes bland and usually serves as drinks in summer time.

Instant Granules (Chong Ji) is prepared by incorporating aqueous herbal extract with sugar, starch or paste and dried to form granules. The granules can be taken instantly when dissolved in hot water. It is a more convenient preparation than decoction and is widely used. It should be stored in sealed packets to prevent from dampness.

Injection (*Zhen Ji*) is a bacterial free, sterilised solution obtained by extracting and refining ingredients from herbs. It is used for subcutaneous or intramuscular and intravenous injections. It has the characteristics of being accurate in dosage, quick in action, convenient to use and of not being affected by food and digestive juice. Examples are Injectio Bupleuri, Injectio Salviae Miltiorrhizae, Injectio San Mai San (Note: The use of injection containing herbal mixture is allowed in China by doctors of TCM but is not practised in other countries unless certain conditions are fulfilled).

CONCLUSION

In conclusion, for TCM treatment with herbal prescriptions, a good command of the knowledge of TCM herbs in common use, theory and method of prescription (Fu Fang Xue) including modification of prescriptions (Fu Fang), and knowledge of dosage forms is required of the TCM practitioner. Thus in writing out a TCM prescription not only the established principles should be followed, modifications must also be made flexibly for individual cases by using the correct dosage form in order to reduce harmful effects and achieve the desired therapeutic goals. Various commonly used prescriptions have been prepared as ready-made TCM patent products commercially available. These are listed out and presented in the Appendix Section as 101 items. However, readers should consult the references in Chapter 4 for examples of well-known prescriptions. Moreover, readers should be aware of the fact that quality of these products is not uniformly controlled in many countries. Most current practice of prescribing TCM herbs depends on how well trained the TCM practitioners are. TCM pharmacists dispense the prescriptions and the patients are advised with instructions for preparing the decoctions.

REFERENCES

Readers should consult the general reference list in Chapter 4 for information. In addition the following references may be useful.

Ou Ming (1991) *Chinese-English Manual of Common-used Prescriptions in Traditional Chinese medicine.* GuangDong Science and Technology Press, GuangDong, China. ISBN: 7-5359-0872-1/R.

The Pharmacopoeia Commission of PRC (1992) *Pharmacopoeia of the People's Republic of China.* GuangDong Science and Technology Press, GuangDong, China. English Edition, ISBN: 7-5359-0945-O/R 174.

Section Two

Interactions Between Chinese Herbal Medicinal Products and Orthodox Drugs

6. OBSERVATIONS OF THE USE OF CHINESE HERBAL MEDICINAL PRODUCTS AND ORTHODOX DRUGS

KELVIN CHAN

THE USE OF TRADITIONAL CHINESE MEDICINE WITH ORTHODOX MEDICAL PRACTICE IN SOME FAR EAST COMMUNITIES

In China, since 1949 the government has re-addressed the importance of traditional Chinese medicine (TCM) practice for the nation's healthcare programmes in parallel with orthodox medicine(OM). The organisation that is responsible for public health that encompass TCM, OM, medical apparatus, scientific research and education is the State Council who empowers the Ministry of Public Health (MPH) to be in charge of these disciplines. The MPH provides two unique health systems in China. About 60% of healthcare are provided by OM and 40% by TCM. Provision of OM and TCM medications is the responsibility of the State Pharmaceutical Administration (SPAC) and the State Administration of TCM (SATCM) respectively. The Government's policy of integration of the two health providers into one system reflects that about 80% of medications used in the rural areas is estimated to be Chinese herbal medicinal (CHM) products. One of the reasons is because CHM products are more economical and thus an important means of cost saving to the Government. The TCM Division of the Ministry of Public of Health (MPH), SATCM, which also controls the practice of TCM, monitors all academic courses of TCM in universities and colleges. In each of the 23 provinces, 3 major municipalities (Beijing, Shanghai and Tianjin), and 5 autonomous regions there is at least one research institute of TCM which is linked with local TCM hospitals for manufacturing, practice, education and research of various disciplines of TCM. Most hospitals are equipped with both orthodox and TCM pharmacies. Some hospitals have integrated departments with specialists in both TCM and orthodox medicine. Patients can choose either treatment. In orthodox hospitals, TCM outpatient departments are available for consultation. The supply of crude herbs and manufacturing of TCM products are controlled by the 'Provisions for New Drug Approval' (1992) issued by the MPH via the SATCM. The most important functions of the SATCM are: (1) to develop and implement Government policy for the industry, including medium to long term plan and annual plan, (2) to ensure the regulations are enforced, (3) to handle financial management including funding projects relating to industrial development, (4) to monitor overall production of CHM medicaments and preparations, and (5) to develop the profiles of the TCM industry abroad and international co-operation. Pharmacies and drug-stores in local areas provide the over-the-counter (OTC) sale of both CHM and OM medications to the public according to regulations set up by the MPH via the SATCM. Most TCM remedies and OM drugs can be purchased as OTC without a prescription with the exception of substances with specific addictive or toxic actions (Chan, 1996).

In Taiwan, after the Second World War and under American influence the practice of orthodox medicine has been the main stream of healthcare although TCM was still practised and used by some of the populace. But as people have become wealthier and the access to OM has improved there has been a continued drift away from TCM. This is particularly obvious among the young who now have higher pressure from jobs. Many of those in their 20s and 30s believe TCM treatment is too slow to get them well from illnesses. Yet the trading of Chinese herbal medicinal (CHM) products and raw herbs in so many herbal shops has maintained good business. This is because the vast majority of the turnover is for tonic herbs such as Dang Gui, Huang Qi, Qou Qi Zi,Ren shen, etc. which many Taiwanese families use in cooking soups and stews particularly in winter seasons. Moreover, women after giving birth, patients after major surgical operations and the elderly would consume CHM herbs to recuperate their strength. It was only until the early 1990s that virtually all health care OM or TCM was private, either paid for directly by the individual or through insurance scheme that cover both OM and TCM treatment.

During the late 1980s the Taiwanese government decided to rationalise the quality and standard of TCM practice and CHM products by setting up a special national examination to screen the existing TCM practitioners for their competence of practice and control on quality of CHM medications. The control on the quality of the TCM practitioners and the manufacturing and provision of the CHM products is the Special Committee of TCM under the administrative power of the Executive Yuan (Council) of the Ministry of Health in Taipei. Before the national examination most of the TCM practitioners obtain their experience from generation before them although some were properly trained at the only TCM College in Tai Chung. After passing the special examination with 18 months practice training at the China Medical College in Taichung all the older generation TCM practitioners can practise under the new national health scheme. Presently, patients in Taiwan can choose to be treated by OM of TCM practitioners. Many CHM product manufacturers in Taiwan have Good Manufacturing Practice guidelines for these products.

In Hong Kong, there has not been any legal restriction on the practice of TCM throughout the whole history of the British colonial period. Until the early 1990s he Department of Health have made initiatives by organising Working Parties, consisting of various professionals, to look at the regulation of TCM products since 1991 and the rationalisation of the qualification of TCM practitioners since 1995. Recently, the Research Grant Council has given substantial amount of funding for research and development of TCM in Hong Kong even though biomedical science research and other physical sciences have always taken the lion share of the research funding. About 70% of the patient population have enjoyed their own self-medication and over 50% consult private TCM practitioners to supplement their speedy need for recovery from illnesses (Working Party Report, 1991). In the Report, which was set out to obtain unbiased observation of how patients respond to their illnesses, it is interesting to note that, major problems with OM and TCM have rarely been reported. TCM practitioners are consulted much less often than OM doctors and only on certain chronic diseases or desparate cases. Children are rarely taken to TCM practitioners. There is strong support for legal regulation for TCM practitioners and less extent, for CHM products (Chan, 1996).

In Japan, orthodox medical doctors who have received training in Kampo medicine (an oriental medicine with modified TCM approaches) can prescribe Kampo treatment and medications of TCM composite formulae. Research and development of Kampo medicinal products has been very advance in particular the areas of composite formulae used in ancient Chinese prescriptions. Many patients have consulted Kampo practitioners as part of their healthcare programmes (Chan, 1996).

THE INFLUENCE OF TRADITIONAL CHINESE MEDICINE IN ORTHODOX MEDICAL PRACTICE IN NON-CHINESE CULTURE

The public in the West has expressed both interests and concerns on the use and practice of TCM. It is a holistic system of medicine with its own philosophy, method of diagnosis and treatments using acupuncture and related physical therapies as well as an unique system of materia medica. The recent successful control, using a TCM composite prescription consisting of 10 herbs in the form of an aqueous decoction, of atopic eczema that has been resistant to orthodox treatment, has created greater interest and attention on the use of TCM herbs and treatment in Britain (Rustin and Poulter, 1996). At present, the quality, efficacy, and safety of these treatment and medicines is uncertain in the West. It will be useful to note how TCM practice has been initiated in Europe, to compare with the progress of this discipline in the Far East and to forecast its future development in health care.

Early knowledge of acupuncture and TCM hebalism in European culture was mainly through returning merchants of the Dutch and English East India Company. Willem ten Rhyjne compiled the first European text on acupuncture in 1683. In the late 19th century, with European influence in the Far East, China and Indo-China much more knowledge of acupuncture percolated through to the West. J M Church in 1821 published the first extensive British text of acupuncture. The British Acupuncture Association was founded in 1961 by a group of practitioners who studied acupuncture in need for adequate educational and ethical standards. Subsequently the British College of Acupuncture was set up in 1964 and other schools and professional societies were set up in the 1970s, 1980s and recently. At present there are five registers of acupuncture and related TCM herbalism and eight schools offering acupuncture and TCM herbalism in various parts of UK. Most of them offer 2 to 4 years part time courses with certificates or diplomas on graduation (Jin et al., 1995). The Register of Chinese Herbal Medicine and the recently established Council for Acupuncture (from the previous Directory of British Acupuncturists in 1982) with five professional associations in 1994 indicated the profession's intention to work to maintain common standards of professionalism in the practice of TCM in the UK.

The number of privately run schools of TCM or related oriental medicine, mainly involved with tuition of acupuncture practice, has increased from several since 1985 to more than ten by the early 1990s. The number of TCM clinics with acupuncture therapy has also increased rapidly in major UK cities, mainly in London, from 600 to nearly approximately 1000 by mid 1990s. Although acupuncture has been the main practice of TCM in these clinics for pain relief and other chronic illnesses most practitioners also prescribed CHM herbal prescriptions with instructions for preparing decoction or ready made CHM products. These products are, mainly supplied by two to three major TCM import and re-export herbal companies, imported from various sources abroad with no legal restriction at present. Evidently patients have taken these preparations as part of their treatment. No study has been reported for the likely herb-drug interactions. But reports on toxicity of CHM treatment mainly concerned with certain CHM products that cause liver and kidney toxicity with occasional cases of heavy metal intoxication. (Graham-Brown, 1992). Several cases of toxicity of CHM herbs have been related to the use of wrong herbs (Atherton, et al, 1993). On the academic side, currently two university courses are being run in acupuncture in the UK. A 5-year course with similar curriculum as that of TCM universities in China has been launched in one of the British universities, in response to public demand on quality of such medical practice. However more comprehensive systems to control both the practice and products may be necessary in the West in order to gain confidence of TCM.

Quite separately, the development of TCM or related Oriental practice in other developed countries such as Australia, Canada, France, Germany, Japan and the USA has taken a noticeable step (Chan and Lee, 2000). It is evident that the possibility of patients' taking CHM medications and OM drugs is pretty high in the future.

THE IMPORTANCE OF MASTERING THE USE AND INTERACTIONS OF CHINESE HERBAL MEDICINAL PRODUCTS AND ORTHODOX DRUGS

It is obvious that in the coming 21st century, people will be more informed about medical products and knowledgeable about matters relating to their health in curing and preventing illnesses. They may demand good quality treatment from both orthodox as well as other complementary medicine. The future professionals in medical care should be knowledgeable on their patients' medications to be aware of possible treatment interactions as they may be given both treatments intentionally or unintentionally, with or without the awareness of the practitioner.

It is observed that patients in the Far East intentionally or unintentionally may be prescribed Chinese herbal medicinal (CHM) products and orthodox medical (OM) preparations for alleviating their illnesses. There are practices of incorporating OM drugs into CHM preparations. The rationale may be that it is hoped to reduce side effects of OM drugs, or to produce synergistic effects for better treatment outcome. It has become apparent that not many of these combinations are successful. Some of the over-the-counter CHM products containing OM drugs are available to the public. In most cases the pharmacological mechanisms of the combinations are not well studied and exaggerated adverse effects or therapeutic failures have been observed. Patients may also self-medicate with CHM tonic preparations while being treated with OM drugs. When several OM drugs are taken together, drug-drug interactions with detrimental effects occur (refer to Chapter 3) and the situation becomes more complicated when CHM products are taken simultaneously. In the West, apart from the Chinese communities, non-Chinese ethnic patients will definitely be exposed to CHM medications through increasing popularity. The problems of herb-drug interactions will exist. Therefore adverse reactions consequential to CHM products may not be as simple as those due allegedly to toxicity of the herbs only.

The concept of integrating the practice of traditional Chinese medicine (TCM) into orthodox medicine (OM) in China has given the opportunity to look at the advantages and disadvantages of each practice and take the benefit from each discipline in order to encourage improvement of healthcare and possibly save treatment costs. China is the only country in the world that has developed a healthcare system that has incorporated traditional medicine into the healthcare policy for the nation. Within the system the two forms of medical treatment work along side with each other at every level of the healthcare structure. In particular, patients can benefit from preventive medicine, reducing side effects from OM or TCM medications and improved quality of life in terminal cases. To achieve these goals it will take a lot of understanding from professionals of both disciplines. No longer should practitioners from TCM and OM be working in isolation. Professionals who are supportive of this concept of integration should also work to find out if there is any benefit at all in combination treatments. Augmenting OM with acupuncture has been recognised in several areas of pain relief, drug dependence etc. in the West. This Chapter only concerns with herb-drug interactions relating to beneficial outcomes or adverse reactions as a consequence of co-administration.

In China, increasing attention has turned towards organised scientific research on this aspect of interactions with beneficial outcomes. From the diet and nutrition aspects many Chinese patients in the community often self medicate with tonic CHM products after serious illnesses or surgical operations while they are still on OM medications. They believe that the herbs will help them to recover rapidly. It is normal procedure to carry out diagnosis of the same patient using TCM procedures and OM modern instruments and techniques in hospital practice in China. Experienced TCM and or OM practitioners who are knowledgeable of using both types of medications have prescribed both types for certain diseases in order to get effective treatments. The improvement or deterioration of patients' disease conditions is the measurement of success or failure of treatment. Some of the observations have been published, mainly in Chinese, in medical journals available in China. Chapter 7 summarises these in table forms.

REFERENCES

Atherton, D. J. Rustin, M.H.A. and Brostoff, J.(1993) Need for correct identification of herbs in poisoning. *Lancet*, **341**, 637–638.

Chan, K. (1996) Critical assessment of traditional Chinese medicine. A Fellowship Report submitted to the Winston Churchill Memorial Trust, London, April 1996.

Chan, K. (1997) Bridging the gap between east and west in the understanding of biomedical sciences of Chinese medicine. An Inaugural Professorial Lecture, Middlesex University, London, *North Cicular*, **75**, 3.

Chan, K. and Lee, H. (2000) *The Way Forward for Traditional Chinese Medicine*, Harwood, Amsterdam. In preparation.

Graham-Brown, R. (1992) Toxicity of Chinese Herbal remedies. *Lancet*, **340**, 673.

Jin, Y., Berry, M.I. and Chan, K. (1995) Chinese herbal medicine in the U.K., *Pharmaceutical Journal*, **255** (suppl.), R37.

Rustin, M.H.A. and Poulter, L. (1996) Chinese herbal therapy in atopic dermatitis. *Dermatological Therapy*, **1**, 83–93.

Working Party Report, (1991) The utilisation of traditional Chinese medicine in Hong Kong. *An Interim Report*, Hong Kong Government Printer, Hong Kong.

7. EXAMPLES OF INTERACTIONS BETWEEN CHINESE HERBAL MEDICINAL PRODUCTS AND ORTHODOX DRUGS

LILY CHEUNG AND KELVIN CHAN

INTRODUCTION

For writing up this particular Section of the book the authors have reviewed information concerning CHM herb-drug interactions reported in medical and scientific literature available in Chinese language. Most of these journals and texts come from research institutes and universities in China. This Chapter is divided into two parts. 'Part One' deals with consequences of interactions leading to beneficial effects while 'Part Two' gives examples of adverse reactions. These observations are given either in Case Study formats or in Tables. References to these publications are given immediately next to the text or tables for easy access. These interactions are selected according to their importance of clinical observations with case studies. Some of the observations have been reported in several journals from different hospitals in different provinces in China. The journals and texts chosen are of recognised sources with good reputation.

When the information is given in Case Study format, information on the Author(s), Title, and Journal of the publication is presented as a 'Heading' followed by a summary of the study, OM drugs and CHM medications involved and suggested mechanisms of interactions. When appearing in Table form the information is organised with headings such as Herbs, Ready-made Medicines, Orthodox Drugs, Reason (of interaction), Result and References. Each of the herbs is referred to its Chinese Pin Yin name, Latin name, and Chinese characters. Similarly for each ready-made medicine these names are also mentioned. All the numbered references are presented at the end of the Chapter as specific references. Tables 7.1 to 7.16 summarise the compiled herb-drug interactions showing adverse effects.

PART ONE: CONSEQUENCES OF HERB-DRUG INTERACTIONS LEADING TO BENEFICIAL EFFECTS

Possible Mechanisms of Beneficial Herb-Drug Interactions

In the integral treatment of illnesses using TCM and OM medications the aim is to bring together the general concepts of syndrome differentiation of TCM with the OM principles of disease differentiation. It is obvious that the two systems vary greatly in approaches of diagnosis and treatment. For instance, OM concerns with microcosmic differentiation of disease state, quantitative analysis of regional lesions or tissues damages, distinction between different disease based on characteristics of pathogenic factors and pathology of lesions. TCM on the other hand, deals with macrocosmic differentiation of syndrome, comprehensive qualitative analysis of whole body, distinction between different syndromes based on complex responses to external and internal pathogenic factors. It is logical to combine observations from disease differentiation (OM) and syndrome differentiation (TCM) of the patient in order to draw accurate diagnostic conclusion. Treatment can be derived to target regional lesion or misfunction (OM) and imbalance holistic conditions (TCM) of the patient. This is one of the principles for integral treatment based on TCM and OM. Modern medical technology and sophistication will help to make OM differential diagnosis while experience and personal approaches is needed for accurate TCM diagnosis. It is necessary to relate the relationship of TCM principles of *Yin* and *Yang* balance of the body to the OM understanding of the inter-play between the body's nervous-endocrine-immune regulation.

Examples of some integral approaches, resulting in beneficial treatment observation and outcomes, are suggested as probable explanation or possible mechanisms of interactions although more experimental research and clinical evidences are needed to confirm such observations. The following tentative categories of case studies illustrate synergy effects of treatment consequential to co-administration of OM drugs and Chinese herbal medicinal (CHM) products. These case studies were abstracted from medical journals published in China and have been translated into English and edited by the authors for presentation in the text.

Category 1   Co-administrating antibiotics with CHM products producing added beneficial effects

Case Study 1   Luo, R-D. (1982). Trimethoprim (TMP) and Shui Yang Mei (*Adinarubella*) in Treating Typhoid. *Chinese Journal of Modern Developments in Traditional Medicine*, **2**(4), 246.

In 33 cases, patients were given 30ml of CHM decoction Shui Yang Mei (orally 3 times a day) plus TMP (0.1g, twice daily) for treating the typhoid. In the control group, 21 patients were given Sulfamethoxazole (SMZ; 1G) and TMP (0.1g), twice daily for the same infection. Both groups of patients were all fully recovered with no recurrence. The curative effects of the two groups were mostly identical (P > 0.05). But the CHM-TMP group had no noticeable side effects. From laboratory experimental evidence, 10% Shui Yang Mei aqueous solution showed bacteriostasis to Shigella dysenteriae. This combined CHM-OM medication showed synergic effect on Salmonella typhia.

Case Study 2   Wu, Y. C. (1984) Treatment of acute bacillary dysentery with traditional Chinese medicine and western medicine combined, on analysis of 117 cases. *Chinese Journal of Integrated and Western Medicine*, **4**(9), 525.

The 117 patients with acute bacillary dysentery were divided into 3 different treatment groups, orthodox medication, OM only, sulfamethoxazole (**SMZ 40 patients**), Chinese herbal medicinal, CHM, prescription 1 (**CHM 1, 36 patients**), and OM plus CHM prescription 2 (**SMZ plus CHM2, 41 patients**). CHM prescription 1 consisted of 10 CHM herbs: Bai Shao (*Radix Paeoniae Alba*), Bai Tou Weng (*Radix Pulsatillae*), Chi Shao (*Radix Paeoniae Rubra*), Da Fu Pi (*Pericarpium Arecae*), Da Huang (*Radix et Rhizoma Rhei*), Dang Gui (*Radix Angelicae Sinensis*), Huang Lian (*Rhizoma Coptidis*), Huang Qin

(*Radix Scutellariae*), Mu Xiang (*Radix Aucklandiae*) and Qin Pi (*Cortex Fraxini*). CHM prescription 2 consisted of 10 CHM herbs: Bai Zhu (*Rhizoma Atractylodis Macrocephalae*), Bai Shao (*Radix Paeoniae Alba*), Bing Lang (*Semen Arecae*), Chi Shao (*Radix Paeoniae Rubra*), Dang Gui (*Radix Angelicae Sinensis*), Fu Ling (*Poria*), Huang Qin (*Radix Scutellariae*), Mu Xiang (*Radix Aucklandiae*),Shan Yao (*Rhizoma Dioscoreae*) and Sheng Jun (*Radix et Rhizoma Rhei*). Four herbs were common in both CHM prescriptions.

Treatment outcomes indicated that the combination medication gave the best results than either of the two groups with single medication treatment (P < 0.005). Comments from the publication are: the SMZ had strong bacteriostatic action that often leads to disproportionate population of intestinal bacteria and dysfunction of the stomach and intestine. The CHM medication is not only free of side effects, it can also increase the body defence mechanism by enhancing the release of immunological factors, phagocytosis of reticuloendothelial system, and by activating the kinase system it increases the amount of bateriophages in acute bacillary dysentery.

Case Study 3   Liu, J-S. (1985). Penicillin, streptomycin and Chinese herbs in treating mastitis. *Chinese Journal of Modern Developments in Traditional Medicine*, **5**(6), 370.

In 68 cases of early mastitis, 34 cases were treated using antibiotics only and the remaining 34 cases were given antibiotics and herbal decoction. The antibiotics group received intramuscular injections, twice daily, of penicillin (800,000 μ) and streptomycin (0.5 g) for 5 days. In addition to the antibiotics used above, aqueous decoction of heat clearing and detoxicating herbs was co-administered orally, daily for 5 days. These herbs included: Jin Yin Hua, *Flos Lonicerae*, 30g; Pu Gong Ying, *Herba Taraxaci*, 30g; Yu Jin, *Radix Curcumae*, 10g; Lou Lu, *Radix Rhapontici*, 12g; Chi Sha, *Radix Paeoniae Rubra* 12g; Qing Pi, *Pericarpium Citri Reticulatae Viride*, 10g; Dan Shen, *Radix Salviae Miltiorrhizae*, 20g; Tong Cao, *Medulla Tetrapanacis*, 8g. In the antibiotics group, 12 cases (35.3%) claimed full recovery, 3 cases (8.8%) showed improvement and 19 cases (55.9%) has no improvement. In the antibiotic-herbal group, 30 cases (88.2%) were fully recovered, 2 cases (5.9%) were improved and 2 cases (5.9%) had no improvement. The total effective rate was 94.1%. Thus, the curative effect of the combination treatment was significantly better (P < 0.001).

Case Study 4   Xu, Y-Z. (1987). Reduction of side effects of Streptomycin by Gan Cao (*Radix Glycyrrhizae*). *Chinese Journal of Modern Developments in Traditional Medicine*, **3**(7), 137.

It is well known that streptomycin can cause damage to the VIIIth cranial nerve and lead to sensorineural deafness. This toxicity of streptomycin was reduced when it was co-administered with Gan Cao. About 80% of the patients who previously were not able to tolerate the side effects persisted in streptomycin treatment.

Case Study 5   Jun, L-R. (1989). Enhancement of Ampicillin action by Shan Zha (*Fructus Crataegi*). *Chinese Journal of Modern Developments in Traditional Medicine*, **4**(9), 315.

The anti-bacterial activity of ampicillin was enhanced in acid urine. Oral administration of decoction of Shan Zha (500 ml, t.i.d.) could maintain urinary acidic at the pH range of 4.5 to 5.5. The bactericidal action of ampicillin against Escherichia coli and Streptococcus faecalis was 10 times stronger at acidic urine than in alkaline urine.

Case Study 6   Liu, J-B. (1993). Reduction of side effects due to Furadantin by Gan Cao (*Radix Glycyrrhizae*) *Shandong Journal of Traditional Chinese Medicine*, **6**(12), 37.

Furadantin has a potent effect on both Gram's positive and negative bacteria, but it causes gastrointestinal disturbance. Concomitant administration of Gao Cao significantly reduced furadantin's adverse reactions and relieved the gastrointestinal symptoms while its anti-bacterial effect was not altered.

Category 2.   Combating infection with antibiotics and immune-strengthening CHM herbs

It is feasible to kill off bacterial infection in the body using OM antibiotics (i.e. OM's regional lesions) while reinforce the body immuno-function using CHM herbs to strengthen the body defence system (i.e. TCM holistic approach). The body's immune system recognises and destroys substances foreign to the body, including bacterial cells, other micorbes, and foreign toxic compounds. Cells in the circulatory and the lymphatic systems that recognise and destroy these cells are generated in the bone marrow and the lymphatic tissue (thymus, lymph nodes, spleen and tonsils), respectively. These 'stem cells' when initially produced are featureless and cannot be distinguished as what type of blood cells (erythrocytes or different kinds of white blood cells) they will become. After their release into the blood stream they are delivered to all parts of the body. Some become 'memory cells' that as the name implies, recognise specific foreign cells or chemicals to which they have been exposed, and react immediately on the next encountering of those compounds. Substances, such as vaccines, that effect the 'memory cells' stimulate only to one disease or antigen. In general, most herbs that contain so many different chemical compounds, for the immune system do not affect 'memory cells', but are general immune system stimulators or immunostimulants. They induce the activities of the immune system but are not specific to a particular disease or antigen (i.e. the protein against which immune cells act). They increase resistance by mobilising 'effector cells' that act against all foreign particles, rather than one specific type. Thus the combination of OM antibiotics with CHM products for treating infectious diseases is a logical approach. This may help to reduce bacterial resistance to antibiotics.

Huang Qi alone is used as a tonic herb and as medicinal herb in combination with others for strengthening the *Lung* for frequent colds or shortness of breath. It has no demonstrable anti-bacterial effects but it increases the immune system by increasing the number of 'stem cell' in bone marrow and lymph tissues, promoting immune cells from the 'resting' state into heightened activity and reducing the negative side effects of co-administered steroids on the immune system. Quite a few of the CHM products in the form of established Ready-made medications or well-tried prescriptions have been shown to possess immuno-strenghtening or modulating properties (see examples in Category 5).

Category 3.   Augmenting cardiovascular OM treatment with CHM products

The beta-adrenergic blocker, propranolol, has been co-administered with aqueous extract of Dan Shen (*Radix Salviae Miltiorrhzae*) as intravenous injection for treating patients suffering acute myocardial-infarction in Intensive Care Coronary Unit in some hospitals in China. The combination treatment gives significantly better outcomes than propranolol alone. Dan Shen aqueous extracts, among many other pharmacological properties, increase microcirculation, inhibit platelet aggregation and have centrally acting anti-anxiety actions.

These may explain the beneficial effects on propranolol. Extensive research works have been carried out over the past 15 years on Dan Shen in Shanghai and Hong Kong academic research institutes. Isolated single chemical entities from Dan Shen roots have not produced any useful and marketable conventional drugs. Apart from injectables other oral preparations of single herb or composite formulae of Dan Shen are available to the public as preventive remedies against cardiovascular diseases. If these products are not used properly, adverse reactions may result if taken with other OM medications (refer to Part 2 of this Chapter).

Category 4. Augmenting anti-inflammatory action of OM drugs with CHM Products

Case Study 1   Ruan, J. and Ye, R.G. (1994) Lupus nephritis treated with impact therapy of cyclophosphamide and traditional Chinese medicine. *Chinese Journal of Integrated Traditional and Western Medicine*, 5(14), 276.

Seventy-six patients suffering from lupus nephritis were divided into two treatment groups, OM medication with cyclophosphamide and steroid (35 patients) and combined OM treatment with CHM decoction of 14 herbs (41 patients). The 14 CHM herbs were, Bai Hua She She Cao (*Herba Heyotis Diffusae*), Ban Zhi Lian (*Herba Scutellariae Barbatae*), Dan Pi (*Cortex Moutan Radicis*), Fu Ling (*Poria*), Han Lian Cao (*Herba Eclipitae*), Ju Hua (*Flos Chrysanthemi*), Nu Zhen zi (*Fructus Ligustri Lucidi*), Qi Zi (*Fructus Lycii*), Shan Yao (*Rhizoma Dioscoreae*), Shan Zhu Yu (*Fructus Corni*), Shu Di (*Radix Rehmanniae Preparata*), Wu Gong (*Scolopendra*), Wu Shao She (*Zaocys*) and Ze Xie (*Rhizoma Alismatis*).

After a six-month treatment course, the therapeutic efficacy was significantly higher in the combination group than the OM medication only group (P<0.05). Cyclophosphamide itself is inactive; after oral administration it is metabolised to active metabolites. In OM prednisone (coticosteroid) is often used together in order to increase the rate of metabolism of cyclophosphamide; although single doses of the steroid will inhibit activation of this potent immunosuppressant. Cycolphosphamide, itself causes liver toxicity and long term steroid treatment also causes systemic side effects. The use of CHM herbs may help to build up beneficial effects by rectifying the imbalance of the body functions according to TCM concepts. Lupus nephritis usually manifests itself as *Liver-Kidney Yin Xu* (deficiency) with symptoms such as, lassitude of the loin and legs, dizziness, tinnitus, dry mouth and throat, deep and small pulse, red tongue with a little coating etc. The CHM herbs in the decoction nourish the *Liver* and *Kidney, Yin* and clear away *Heat*.

Case 2   Ye, R. G. *et al.* (1993) Observation on 134 patients with adult primary nephrotic syndrome with combined traditional Chinese medicine and Western medicine treatment. *Chinese Journal of Integrated Traditional and Western Medicine*, 13(2), 84.

The 134 patients suffering adult primary nephrotic syndrome were separated randomly into two groups and treated with corticosteroid (66 patients) and steroid with a decoction consisting of 10 herbs (68). The 10 CHM herbs were, Dan Shen (*Radix Salviae Miltiorrhzae*), Di Gu Pi (*Cortex Lycii Radicis*) Gui Ban (*Plastrum Testudinis*), Han Lian Cao (*Herba Ecliptae*) Hong Hua (*Flos Carthami*), Nu Zhen Zi (*Fructus Ligustri Lucidi*), Qi Zi (*Fructus Lycii*), Sheng Di (*Radix Rehmanneae*), Yi Mu Cao (*Herba Leonuri*) and Zhi Mu (Rhizoma Anemarrhenae).

The percentage of success from the corticosteroids treatment and the combined therapy was 56.1% and 85.3% respectively and the corresponding percentages for incidence of side effects were 48% and 14.8%. These observations indicate that corticosteroid plus

CHM decoction could enhance curative success with fewer side effects.

Category 5.   Reducing adverse effects due to OM chemotherapy during treatment of cancers by CHM products

Chemotherapeutic treatment of cancers (malignant neoplasm or new growth) is often started after not so successful of, or in conjunction with, radiation therapy. At this late stage patients become physically weak with quite a few signs of adverse effects as the treatment used often affects normal cells. The most severe toxic effects include bone marrow suppression, and nausea and vomiting apart from impairment of healing, depression of growth, causing sterility and hair loss. Some patients become in tolerable to chemotherapy and their quality of life is much reduced. Their immune system is highly compromised. Cytotoxic drugs for cancer treatment, depending on which cancer types and the policy for chemotherapy, often consists of at least three and more different groups of anti-neoplamsic agents. They are anti-metabolites (cytarabine, fluorouracil, methotrexate, and mercaptopurine), cytotoxic antibiotics (bleomycin, dactinomycin, doxurubicin, epirubicin, and mitomycin), plant derivatives (etoposide, vincristine), hormones and their antagonists (glucocorticoid, oetrogens such as fosfestrol, anti-oestrogen such as tamoxifen, progestrogens such as megestrol, anti-androgen antagonists such as cyproterone and flutamide, and gonadotrophin-releasing hormone such as goserelin, radio-isotopes such as ^{131}I for thyroid tumours and inhibitors of DNA and RNA (procarbazine).

Chemotherapy treatment of cancers using integral approach of OM and CHM herbs has been practised in some hospitals in China. The concept is to utilise OM cytotoxic agents to target the cancerous cells and CHM medications for restoring imbalances, as diagnosed from clinical picture, due either to the neoplasm or chemotherapy. The following cases illustrate some of the observations.

Case Study 1   Rao, X. Q. Yu. R. C. *et al.* (1990) Clinical and experimental studies on chemotherapy combined with "Sheng Xue Tang" (SXT) recipe for the treatment of late stage gastric cancer. *Beijing Journal of Traditional Chinese Medicine (China),* (**1**), 46–49.

Eighty-one late-stage gastric cancer patients were treated with chemotherapy (MFV, methotrexate, Fluorouracil, vinblastin; or MFC, methotrexate, fluorouracil, combinations). Among them, 63 patients also took the herbal recipe SXT while other 18 patients were treated with chemotherapy only as control group. The recipe included following eight herbs: *Radix Astragalus*; *Radix Pseudostellariae*; *Caulis Spatholobi*; *Rhizoma Atyractylodis Macrocephalae*; *Poria*; *Fructus Lycii*; *Fructus Ligustri Lucidi* and *Semen Cuscutae*. Clinical observations showed that the recipe could reduce the side effects caused by chemotherapy with improved body weight (see following summaries).

A summary of adverse effects during chemotherapy treatment with and without SXT recipe.

Groups	Chemotherapy plus SXT recipe 33 cases (100%)	Chemotherapy only (control) 12 cases (100%)
Loss of appetite	12 (19%)	6 (50%)
Nausea and Vomiting	12 (19%)	6 (50%)
Diarrhoea	0	6 (50%)
Tiredness	20 (31%)	8 (67%)

Limp numbness	0	4 (33%)

A summary of changes in patients' body weight (kg) during chemotherapy treatment with and without SXT recipe.

Groups	Chemotherapy plus SXT recipe	Chemotherapy only (control)
Number of cases	29	12
Before treatment (X ± SD)	58.51 ± 1.85	58.73 ± 5.53
After treatment (X ± SD)	60.66 ± 3.08	57.16 ± 5.66
T value	18.22	0.688
P value	< 0.001	> 0.05

Separate experimental studies provided evidence that the SXT recipe could prolong the life of the S-180 tumour bearing mice undergone chemotherapy. The results appeared to be in accordance with observations found in the clinical studies.

Case Study 2.   Pan, M.J. and Li, Y.H. (1991) Treatment of side effects caused by chemotherapy in 534 cancer patients using Chinese herbal prescriptions. *Chung Kuo Chung His I Cheieh Ho Tsa Chich*, **11**(4), 233–234.

The composite prescription, "Fu Zheng Jian Pi Tang" (FZJPT) in the form of aqueous decoction (literally meaning that the decoction is for rectifying syndromes by nourishing the '*Spleen*'), contained 15 herbs. They were Huang Qi (*Radix Astragalus*); *Radix Codonopsis*; *Rhizoma Atractylodis Macrocephalae*; *Poria*; *Radix Glycyrrhizae*; *Radix Rehmanniae Preparata*; *Fructus Lycii*; *Radix Polygoni Multiflori*; *Rhizoma Polygonati*; *Fructus Ligustri Lucidi*; *Radix Glehniae*; *Caulis Spatholobi*; *Radix Ophiopogonis*; *Semen Euryalis*; *Rhizoma Dioscoreae*. The decoction was given to 534 cancer patients for the treatment of the side effects caused by chemotherapy. The clinical study showed some encouraging results. The following summary shows the occurrence of the side effects in two groups of patients undergone chemotherapy with or without herbal decoction treatment.

A summary of occurrence of side effects during treatment.

Groups	Chemotherapy plus herbal 534 cases (100%)	Chemotherapy only (control) 86 cases (100%)	P Value
Nausea	138 (25.8%)	70 (81.4%)	<0.01
Vomiting	103 (19.2%)	64 (74.4%)	<0.01
Abdominal distension	108 (20.2%)	54 (62.8%)	<0.01
Diarrhoea	39 (7.3%)	20 (23.3%)	<0.01
Stomach haemorrhage	21 (3.9%)	7 (8.1%)	>0.05
Tiredness	113 (21.2%)	72 (83.7%)	<0.01
Leucopenia	182 (34.1%)	65 (75.6%)	<0.01
Anaemia	86 (16.2%)	32 (37.2%)	<0.01
Trichomadesis	24 (4.5%)	25 (29.1%)	<0.01
Liver damage	32 (6.0%)	15 (17.5%)	<0.01
Kidney damage	14 (2.6%)	5 (5.8%)	>0.05
Myocardial damage	7 (1.3%)	8 (9.3%)	<0.05
Immune inhibition	52 (9.7%)	31 (36.0%)	<0.01

Another group of 40 patients was treated with a modified prescription of the one mentioned above. Some new herbs were added to the prescription (FZJPT) in order to replace some of the original herbs according to the changing conditions of individual patients. This group of patients showed better clinical results (see summary below).

A summary of adverse effects during treatment after modification of FZJPT decoction.

Groups	Chemotherapy plus FZJPT 40 cases (100%)	Chemotherapy plus modified FZJPT 40 cases (100%)
Nausea	11 (27.5%)	9 (22.5%)
Vomiting	10 (25.0%)	7 (17.5%)
Abdominal distension	11 (27.5%)	7 (17.5%)
Diarrhoea	5 (12.5%)	4 (10.0%)
Stomach haemorrhage	3 (7.5%)	1 (2.5%)
Tiredness	8 (20.0%)	6 (15.0%)
Leucopenia	14 (35.0%)	12 (30.0%)
Anaemia	9 (22.5%)	7 (17.5%)
Trichomadesis	5 (12.5%)	1 (2.5%)
Liver damage	1 (2.5%)	0 (0.0%)
Kidney damage	0 (0.0%)	0 (0.0%)
Myocardial damage	0 (0.0%)	0 (0.0%)
Immune inhibition	8 (20.0%)	5 (12.5%)

PART TWO: CONSEQUENCES OF HERB-DRUG INTERACTIONS LEADING TO ADVERSE EFFECTS

INTRODUCTION

This part deals with interactions between CHM and OM medications as reported from the literature mainly available in Chinese language. The information has been edited and compiled into 16 Tables (Table 7.1 to Table 7.16). Some clinical observations have been confirmed with experimental investigation. In general the mechanisms described for drug-drug interactions in Chapter 3 are also applicable for the herb-drug interactions as understood from conventional science and medical aspects. Complications arise because of the presence of so many chemical entities in the single herb or in the decoction of the composite formulae, and many of which have not yet be identified.

Possible Mechanisms of Herb-Drug Interactions

Formation of Insoluble Complexes during Absorption Phase Leading to Therapeutic Failure

Some CHM medications whether single herbs or composite prescription decoction or ready-made products contain metal ions that may form insoluble chelates or complexes with OM drugs (Tables 7.1 and Table 7.2). Tannic acid in some CHM medications (Table 7.3) can form insoluble complexes with OM antibiotics and drugs containing tertiary amine-alkaloids and metal ions. Alkaloids in CHM medications (Table 7.4) form precipitates with metal ions in OM drugs. CHM medications containing quercetin (phenols with 5-OH and 4-keto functional groups) can precipitae OM drugs containing aluminium, bismuth, calcium, ferrous, and magnesium ions (Table 7.5). Gan Cao (Radix Glycyrrhizae) interacts with tetracycline group of antibiotics by reduction of their oral absorption (Table 7.12). Yin Chen (*Herba Artemisiae Capillaris*) forms precipitates with quinidine and antagonises chloramphenicol actions (Table 7.16).

Affecting the Transport of Drug Molecules in the Body by CHM Medications Leading to Reduced Effects

Some CHM medications have high contents of acids that will alter the physiological pH and thus affect the transport mechanisms of OM drug molecules leading to reduced actions or physiological precipitation (Table 7.6). Similarly some CHM medications contain alkali that affect the physiological solubility of the OM drugs thus influencing the excretion and transport of OM drugs (Table 7.7).

Affecting Function of OM Diuretics and Body Electrolyte Balance by CHM Medications

Some OM diuretics such as the potassium-sparing group (amiloride, spironolactone, etc.) should not be co-administered with some CHM medications (see Table 7.8). These products contain potassium ions in various forms. Hyperkalaemia may result due to accumulation of the ion from the herbal products and retention from the diuretics.

Destroying Amylase in Some CHM Medications by OM Antibiotics

Amylase contents in some CHM products are active principles that can be destroyed by tertracylines and sulphonamides (Table 7.9).

Destroying glycosides in some CHM Products by OM Acidic Drugs

Glycosides in some CHM products may be the active ingredients that can be destroyed if OM acidic drugs (Ascorbic acid, nicotinic acid, glutamic acid and drugs containing mineral acid components as salts) are administered concurrently (Table 7.10).

Releasing Toxic Cyanide from CHM Medications by OM Drugs

Some CHM herbs, in particular, seeds when co-administered with OM drugs release hydrocyanic acid that inhibits the respiratory centre (Table 7.11).

Affecting Drug Metabolising Enzyme (DME) Systems In The Liver of OM Drugs By CHM Products

CHM single herb or products may modify the metabolic elimination of OM drugs leading to reducing activity (enzyme induction) or increasing activity (enzyme inhibition) of OM drugs. The pharmacokinetics of warfarin is compromised in during co-administration with Dan Shen (*Radix Salvia Miltiorrhiza*) leading to uncontrollable steady state of plasma concentration (Table 7.14). Warfarin is mainly eliminated by the DME system in the liver and has a narrow therapeutic window during clinical treatment when chronic anticoagulation administration is needed. If the steady state is affected haemorrhagic or clotting episodes will occur. The active ingredient of Gan Cao (*Radix Glycyrrhizae*), glycyrrhizin, is an inhibitor of 11 beta-hydroxysteroid dehydrogenase, a major metabolic enzyme of glucocorticoids in the liver. Co-administration of Gan Cao potentiates the action of prednisolone due to enzyme inhibition.

Examples of Interactions between Some Popular CHM Products and OM Drugs

Gan Cao (Radxi Glycyrrhizae) interacts with OM drugs in several aspects

One of the most widely used CHM ingredients in many prescriptions, Gan Cao, interacts with quite a number of different pharmacological classes of drugs with mostly therapeutic failure of the OM treatments. Theses include: causing physiological imbalance of electrolytes resulting in hypokalaemia, reducing efficacy of oral anti-diabetics and insulin, augmenting loss of potassium due to amphotericin, reducing absorption of antibiotics, etc. (Table 7.12).

Ma Huang (Herba Ephedrae) Interacting with OM Drugs in Several Ways

Ma Huang is one of the popular CHM herbs used in prescriptions. Pharmacologically it has stimulant actions of the central nervous system and augments the adrenergic activities. It enhances the effects of digitalis but reduces sedative effects of hypnotics and tranquillisers. It increases effects of adrenergic agonists (Table 7.13).

Dan Shen (Radix Salvia Miltiorrhiza) Interacting with OM Drugs To Produce Adverse and Beneficial Effects

Dan Shen is one of the most popular herbs that possess cardiovascular activities. Right combination with OM drugs result in beneficial therapy (refer to Part 1 Category 3). It and other CHM combination products containing Dan Shen when used together with OM drugs will manifest adverse actions. With warfarin exaggerated prolongation of prothrombin time is observed resulting excessive bleeding in patients who are on chronic treatment with warfarin. Dan Shen itself does not affect prothrombin time. It is likely that the metabolism of warfarin is compromised during Dan Shen treatment. It reduces the efficacy of anti-ulcer drugs due probably to formation of unabsorbable precipitants. Dan Shen may encourage cell growth due possibly to its ability to increase microcirculation. Thus it reduces the therapeutic efficacy of anti-cancer agents (Table 7.14).

Dang Gui (Radix Angelica Sinensis) Interacting with Warfarin

Dang Gui is often used as a tonic herb and consumed in the form of soup prepared with meat. Proprietary over-the-counter Dang Gui capsules are readily available in most health shops. Clinical observations of patients who have been stabilised on warfarin treatment in hospitals after surgical operation experienced exaggerated bleeding during home rest when they ingest Dang Gui soup. This interaction was also demonstrated in laboratory. Dang Gui does not affect single dose or multiple dosing warfarin-pharmacokinetics. However the prothrombin time is prolonged only at steady state of warfarin treatment. Dang Gui itself does not affect prothrombin time (Table 7.15).

REFERENCES

1. Wang Yu Sheng (Ed.), Pharmacology and Application in Chinese Herbs. People's Health Publisher Ltd., Beijing, China, 1983.
   中药药理与应用王浴生主编人民卫生出版社1983
2. Xu Guo Jun (Ed.) Coloured Illustrations of Chinese Traditional and Herbal Drugs. Fu Jian Scientific and Technical Publisher Ltd., 1989.
   中草药彩色图谱 徐国钧福建科学技术出版福1989
3. National Dictionary of Chinese Herbs. Publication Committee. People's Health Publisher Ltd., Beijing, China, 1983.
   全国中草药汇编编写组人民卫生出版社1983
4. Cui Shu De (Ed.), Chinese Herbs Dictionary. Hei Long Jiang Scientific and Technical Publisher Ltd., 1989.
   中药大全崔树德黑龙江科学技术出版社1989
5. Ou Ming, Chinese-English Manual of Common Used Prescriptions in TCM. Joint Publication (H.K.) Co., Ltd., 1989.
6. Gong Li-Rong (1989), Interaction's of Chinese Patent Medicine and Orthodox Drugs (I). Chinese Journal of Integrated Traditional and Western Medicine, **5(9)**, 315–317.
   中成药与西药的相互作用（一）龚丽荣中西医结合杂志1989
7. Gong Li-Rong (1989), Interaction's of Chinese Patent Medicine and Orthodox Drugs (II). Chinese Journal of Integrated Traditional and Western Medicine, **6(9)**, 375–376.
   中成药与西药的相互作用（二）龚丽荣中西医结便杂志1989
8. An Overview on the Combined Use of Chinese Herbs and Orthodox Drugs. Chinese Journal of Integrated Traditional and Western Medicine, 1987, 3(7), 135–138.
   临床中药及中西药联合应用中若干问题的探讨中西医结合杂志1987
9. Xu Rong-Zhao (1984), A Discussion on the Use of Chinese Herbs and Orthodox Drugs. Chinese Journal of Integrated Traditional and Western Medicine, **12(4)**, 756–757.
   谈谈关于中药和西药联合应用的一些问题徐永昭中西医结合杂志1984
10. Mo Xue-sen (1990), The Inhibition Chinese Herbs and Orthodox Drugs. Chinese Journal of Integrated Traditional and Western Medicine, **3(10)**, 187–188.
    中西药联合应用中的配伍禁忌莫学森中西医结合杂志1990
11. Xu Rong-Zhao (1989), Interaction Ma Huang (Herba Ephedrae) and Orthodox Drugs. Chinese Journal of Integrated Traditional and Western Medicine, **4(9)**, 250.
    中药麻黄与西药的相互作用徐永昭中西医结合杂志1989
12. Chan, K (1995), Progress in Traditional Chinese Medicine, Trends in Pharmacological Sciences, **16**, 182–187.
13. Liu Jia-bin (1993), The Combined Use of Chinese Herbs and Orthodox Drugs. Shan Dong Journal of TCM, **6(12)**, 37–38.
    中西药的合理配伍与禁总刘佳彬山东中医杂志1993
14. Li Bin (1990), A Discussion on the Interactions of Chinese Herbs and Antibodics. Shan Dong Journal of TCM, **2(20)**, 28–29.
    谈中西药与抗菌类西药的不合理李彬山东中医杂志1990
15. Zhang Liang-min (1989), A Discussion of the Use of Chinese Herbs and Orthodox Drugs. Shan Dong Journal of TCM, **4(8)**, 38-39
    谈中西药的配伍禁忌张良民山东中医杂志1989
16. Leng Fang-nan (Ed.), Fundamental of Chinese Patent TCM products (I), People's Health Publisher Ltd., Beijing, China, 1988.
    中国基本成药一部冷方南人民卫生出版社1988
17. Leng Fang-nan (Ed.), Fundamental of Chinese patent TCM Products (II), People's Health Publisher Ltd., Beijing, China, 1991.
    中国基本成药一部冷方南人民卫生出版社1991
18. Chan, K, Lo, A.C.T. et al (1995), The Effects of Dan Shen (Salvia Miltiorrhiza) on Warfarin Pharmacodynamics and Pharmacokinetics of Warfarin Enanitimers in Rats. J. Pharm. Pharmacol., **47**, 402–406.
19. Chan, K., Lo, A.C.T. et al (1992), The Effects of Dan Shen (Salvia Miltiorrhiza) on Warfarin Pharmacodynamics and Pharmacokinetics of Warfarin in Rats. European Journal of Drug Metabolism and Phamcokinetics., **17(4)**, 257–262

20. Lo, A.C.T., Chan, K. et al (1995), Dang Gui (Angelica Sinensis) Effects the Pharmacodynamics but not the Pharmacokinetics of Warfarin in Rabbits. European Journal of Drug Metabolism and Pharmacokinetics, **20(1)**, 55–60.

21. Stockley, I.H. (1996) Drug Interactions: A source book of adverse interactions, their mechanisms, clinical importance and management. The Pharmaceutical Press, London.

22. Price List and Catalogue. East West Herbs Ltd., Kingham, Oxfordshire, UK.

23. A Catalogue of Selected Herbs from the Orient and Traditional Chinese Herbal Formulae. May Way UK Ltd., London, UK.

24. The Three Treasures, Giovanni Maciocia, Stock list, East West Herbs Ltd., Kingham, Oxfordshire, UK, 1995.

25. Zhu Jian-hua (Ed.), The Interaction of Chinese Herbs and Orthodox Drugs. People's Health Publisher Ltd., Beijing, China, 1994.
   中西药物相互作用朱建华

26. Jin, Y., Berry, M.I. & Chan, K. (1995), Chinese Herbal Medicine in the United Kingdom. The Pharmaceutical Journal, **225**, R37.

Table 7.1 Interaction between Chinese Medicines Containing Calcium and Orthodox Drugs (Ref. 5, 16, 17, 22, 23, 24)

Herbs	Chinese Medicines — Ready-made Medicines		Orthodox Drugs	Reasons	Results	Ref.
Bai Shao (Radix Pheoniae Alba) 白芍	Ba Zhen Wan	八珍丸	(Tetracyclines)	Calcium and antibiotics will produce precipitation, thus hindering the absorption through the intestinal wall.	Reduces the effect of the antibiotics.	6, 8, 9, 10 13, 14, 15 21 (P111)
Chi Shi Zhi (Halloysitum Rubrum) 赤石脂	Break into a smile	*	(Rolitetracycline Oxytetracycline Aureomycicline, Doxycycline, Declomycine, Minocycline, Methacycline, Demeclocycline) Kanamycin, Neomycin			
Ge Jie (Gecko) 蛤蚧	Bai Hu Tang	白虎汤				
Ge Qiao 蛤壳	Bao He Wan	保和丸				
(Concha Meretrigis Seu Cyclinae)	Bend Bamboo					
Hai Ma (Hippicampus) 海马	Bi Xie Shen Shi Tang	萆解渗湿汤				
Hai Piao Xiao (Os Sepiae) 海螵蛸	Brighten the Eyes	*				
Hua Shi (Talcum) 滑石	Brocade Sinews	*				
Long Chi (Dens Dar-conis) 龙齿	Chai Ge Jie Ji Tang	柴葛解肌汤				
Long Gu (Os Darconis) 龙骨	Chai Hu Shu Gan Tang	柴胡疏肝汤				
Lu Jiao Jiao (Colla Cornus Cervi) 鹿角胶	Chi Feng Zhen Zhu	彩风珍珠暗疮丸				
Lu Jiao Shuang 鹿角霜	An Chuan Wan					
(Cornu Cervi Degelatinatum)	Clear Lustre	*				
Ma Chi Xian (Herba Portulacae) 马齿苋	Da Qing Long Tang	大青龙汤	Digitalis	Both calcium and Digitalis have similar effect of increasing the contraction of cardiac muscle.	Causes Digitalis intoxication and heart arrhythmias.	6, 15 21 (P299) 25 (P173)
Mu Li (Concha Ostreae) 牡蛎	Dang Gui Si Ni Tang	当归四逆汤				
Sang Piao Xiao (Oothecamantidis) 桑螵蛸	Du Huo Ji Sheng Tang	独活寄生汤				
Shan Zha (Fructus Crataegi) 山楂	Fang Feng Tong Sheng San	防风通圣散				
Shi Gao (Gypsum Fibrosum) 石膏						
Shi Jue Ming (Concha Haliotidis) 石决明	Freeing the Moon	*				
Shui Niu Jiao (Cornu Bubali) 水牛角	Gan Mao Ling	感冒灵				

* The samples do not have Chinese names

Table 7.1 *(Continued)*

Herbs	Chinese Medicines		Orthodox Drugs	Reasons	Results	Ref.
	Ready-made Medicines					
Wa Leng Zi (Concha Arcae) 瓦楞子	Gui Zhi Tang	桂枝汤	Isoniazid	Isoniazid contains NHNH2 and will cause precipitation when taken with calcium.	Hinders the absorption of Isoniazid.	6, 9, 10, 13
Zhen Zhu (Margarita) 珍珠	Huang Qi Jian Zhong Tang	黄芪建中汤				
Zhen Zhu Mu (Concha Margaritifera Osta) 珍珠母	Jin Suo Gu Jing Wan	金锁固精丸	Laevodopa	Laevodopa containing phenolic hydroxyl will cause precipitation if taken with calcium.	Reduces biological effect.	6
	Liu Yi San	六一散				
	Ma Xing Shi Gan Tang	麻杏石甘汤				
	Ma Zi Ren Wan	麻子仁丸				
	Ming Mu Di Huang Wan	明目地黄丸				
	Qing Qi Hua Tan Wan	清气化痰丸				
	Ren Shen Yang Rong Wan	人参养荣丸				
	Root the Spirit	*				
	San Huang Shi Gao Tang	三黄石膏汤				
	Shi Chuan Da Bu Wan	十全大补丸				
	Si Ni San	四逆散				
	Si Wu Tang	四物汤				
	Stir Field of Elixir	*				
	Wu Ji Bai Feng Wan	乌鸡白凤丸				
	Xiao Qing Long Tang	小青龙汤				
	Yu Nu Jian	玉女煎				
	Zhen Zhu San	珍珠散				
	Zhu Ling Tang	猪苓汤				
	Zuo Gui Wan	左归丸				

* The samples do not have Chinese names

Table 7.2 Interaction between Chinese Medicines Containing Iron, Magnesium, and Aluminium and Orthodox Drugs (Ref. 5, 16, 17, 22, 23, 24)

Chinese Medicines		Orthodox Drugs	Reasons	Results	Ref.
Herbs	*Ready-made Medicines*				
Containing Iron (Ref. 5, 17, 18, 23, 24, 25)					
Chi Shi Zhi (Halloysitum Rubrum) 赤石脂	Bao He Wan 保和丸	Tetracyclines (Tetracycline, Oxytetracycline, Aureomycline, Doxycline, Declomycine, Minocycline, Methacycline, Demeclocycline)	Precipitation will be caused thus affecting the absorption of the medicine and lowering the serum level.	Reduce antibacterial effect.	6, 8, 9, 10, 13, 15, 21 (P109) 25 (P68, 71, 73)
Ci Shi (Magnetitum) 磁石	Brocade Sinews *				
Dai Zhe Shi (Haematitum) 代赭石	Er Ming Zuo Ci Wan 耳鸣左慈丸				
Ji Xue Teng (Caulis Spatholobi) 鸡血藤	Jin Suo Gu Jing Wan 金锁固精丸				
Long Gu (Os Draconis) 龙骨	Qing Qi Hua Tan Wan 清气化痰丸				
Ma Chi Xian (Herba Portulacae) 马齿苋	Root the Spirit *				
Mu Li (Concha Ostreae) 牡蛎	Wu Ji Bai Feng Wan 乌鸡白凤丸				
Sang Piao Xiao (Oothecamantidis) 桑螵蛸					
Shan Zha (Tructus Crataegi) 山楂					
Zi Ran Tong (Pyritum) 自然铜		Prednisolone	The pharmaceutical strength will be decreased.	Reduce therapeutic effect.	6
Containing Magnesium (Ref. 5, 17, 18, 23, 24, 25)					
Chi Shi Zhi (Halloysitum Rubbum) 赤石脂	Bi Xie Shen Shi Teng 萆薢渗湿汤	Isoniazid	Isoniazid containing NHNH2 will cause precipitation when combined with the metals.	Hinders absorption	6, 9, 10, 13
Hai Piao Xiao (Os Sepiae) 海螵蛸	Liu Yi San 六一散				
Hua Shi (Talcom) 滑石	Root the Spirit *				
Long Gu (Os Draconis) 龙骨	Wu Ji Bai Feng Wan 乌鸡白凤丸				
Lu Jiao Jiao (Colla Cornus Cervi) 鹿角胶	Zhu Ling Tang 猪苓汤				
Lu Jiao Shuang (Cornu Cervi Degelatinatum) 鹿角霜	Zuo Gui Wan 左归丸				
Containing Aluminium (Ref. 5, 17, 18, 23, 24, 25)					
Chi Shi Zhi (Halloysitum Rubbum) 赤石脂	Jin Suo Gu Jing Wan 金锁固精丸	Laevodopa	Precipitation will be formed when Laevodopa consisting of Phenolic Hydroxyl and the metals are taken at the same time.	Reduce biological effect	6
Long Gu (Os Draconis) 龙骨	Root the Spirit *				
Ming Fan (Alumen) 明矾	Wu Ji Bai Feng Wan 乌鸡白凤丸				
Mu Li (Concha Ostreae) 牡蛎					

* The samples do not have Chinese names

Table 7.3   Interaction between Chinese Medicines containing Tannic Acid and Orthodox Drugs (Ref. 5, 16, 17, 22, 23, 24)

Herbs	Medicines		Orthodox Drugs	Reasons	Results	Ref.
	Chinese Medicines					
Bai Jiang Cao (Herba Patriniae)	Ba Zhen Wan	八珍丸	Tetracyclines (Tetracycline,	Precipitation is formed	Hinders absorption and reduce biological effect.	6, 8, 9, 10, 13, 14, 15.
Bai Shao (Radix Paeoniae Alba)	Bai Du San	败毒散	Roletetracycline,			
Ban Zhi Lian (Herba Scutellariae Barbata)	Break into a Smile	*	Oxytetracycline,			
Bi Xie (Rhixoma Dioscoreae Hypoglaucae)	Ban Xia Hou Po Tang	半夏厚朴汤	Aureomycycine,			
	Bao He Wan	保和丸	Doxycycline,			
Bing Lang (Semen Arecae)	Bend Bamboo	*	Declomycine,			
Chi Shao (Radix Paeonia Rubra)	Bi Xie Fen Qing Yin	萆解分清饮	Minocyline,			
Da Fu Pi (Pericarpium Arecae)	Bi Xie Shen Shi Tang	萆解渗湿汤	Methacycline,			
Da Huang (Radix Et Rhizoma Rhei)	Bi Yan Pian	鼻炎片	Demeclocycline)			
Dan Pi (Cortex Moutan)	Brighten the Eyes		Erythromycin,			
Di Gu Pi (Cortex Lycii)	Brucade Sinens		Rifampicin,			
Di Yu (Radix Sanguisorbae)	Bu Zhong Yi Qi Wan	补中益气丸	Griseofulvin,			
Du Zhong (Cortex Eucommiae)	Chai Hu Shu Gan Tang	柴胡疏肝汤	Lincomycin,			
Er Cha (Catecau)	Chi Feng Zhen Zhu An Chuang Wan	彩凤珍珠暗疮丸	Iveomycin,			
Han Lian Cao (Herba Ecliptae)	Chuan Bei Pi Pa Gao	川贝枇杷膏	Chloramphenical			
He Huan Pi (Cortex Albizziae)	Clear Lustre	*	Amoxilline,			
He Zi (Fructus Chebulae)	Clear the Soul		Mycostatin,			
Hou Po (Cortex Magnoliae Officinalis)	Da Bu Yuan Jian	大补元煎	Clindamycin.			
	Da Chai Hu Tang	大柴胡汤				
Hu Zhang (Rhizoma Polygoni Cuspidati)	Da Cheng Qi Tang	大承气汤	Isoniazid,	The herbs, especially He Zi, Wu Bei Zi, Di Yu and the patent medicines containing these herbs are Hepatotoxic. The drugs are also Hepatotoxic. The possibility of toxicity is increased.	Causes hepataotoxic effect.	6, 8, 14.
Huai Hua (Flos Sophorae)	Du Huo Ji Sheng Tang	独活寄生汤	Tetracycline,			
Huai Jiao (Fructus Sophorae)	Er Ming Zuo Ci Wan	耳鸣左慈丸	Rifampin,			
Jin Qian Cao (Herba Lysimachiae)	Fang Feng Tong Sheng San	防风通圣散	Chlorpromazine,			
Kuan Dong Hua (Flos Farfarae)	Freeing the Moon	*	Erythromycin.			
Ma Chi Xian (Herba Portulacae)	Gan Mao Lin	感冒灵				
Mei Gu Hua (Flos Rosae Rugosae)	Ge Xia Zhu Yu Tang	膈下逐瘀汤				
Mu Gua (Fructus Chaenomelis)	Glorious Sea	*				
Pi Pa Ye (Folium Eriobotryae)	Gui Zhi Tang	桂枝汤				

* The samples do not have Chinese names

Table 7.3 (Continued)

Chinese Medicines		Orthodox Drugs	Reasons	Results	Ref.
Herbs	Medicines				
Qi Zi (Fructus Lycii) 杞子	Huang Qi Jian Zhong Tang 黄芪建中汤	Calcium Gluconate, Calcium Carbonate, Aluminium Hydroxide, Atropire, Ferrous Sulphate, Ferri Ammoii Citras, Bismuth Subcarbonate,	The drugs contains metal elements and precipitation will be formed when combining with tannic acid.	Reduces therapeutic effect.	6, 8, 9, 15.
Qian Hu (Radix Peucedani) 前胡	Huo Xiang Zheng Qi Wan 藿香正气丸				
Qing Hao (Herba Artemisaeannuae) 青蒿	Jade Spring *				
Ren Dong Teng (Caulis Lonicerae) 忍冬藤	Jing Fang Bai Du San 荆防败毒散				
Rou Gui (Cortex Cinnamomi) 肉桂	Liu Wei Di Huang Wan 六味地黄丸				
Sang Ye (Folium Mori) 桑叶	Long Dan Xie Gan Tang 龙胆泻肝汤				
Shan Zha (Fructus Crataegi) 山楂	Ma Zi Ren Wan 麻子仁汤				
Shan Zhu Yu (Fructus Corni) 山茱萸	Ming Mu Di Huang Wan 明目地黄丸				
Sheng Ma (Rhizoma Cimmifugae) 升麻	Open the Heart *				
Tu Fu Ling (Rhizoma Smilacis Glabrae) 土茯苓	Ping Wei San 平胃散				
Wei Ling Cai (Hebra Potentillae Cainensis) 委陵菜	Qi Ju Di Huang Wan 杞菊地黄丸	Ephedrine, Strychnine, Quinine, Atpopine, Reserpine, Digitais, Vitamin B1 Antipyrine,	A non-absorbent compound is formed	Reduces therapeutic effect.	6, 8, 9, 10, 13, 15.
Wu Bei Zi (Galla Chinensis) 五倍子	Qing Qi Hua Tan Wan 清气化痰丸				
Wu Jia Pi (Cortex Acanthopanacis) 五加皮	Qing Wei San 清胃散				
Xian He Cao (Herba Agrimoniae) 仙鹤草	Radio Support *				
Xian Mao (Rhizoma Curculiginis) 仙茅	Red Stirring *				
Yin Yang Huo (Herba Epimedii) 淫羊藿	Release Constraint *				
Hu Xing Cao (Herba Houttuyniae) 鱼腥草	Ren Shen Yang Rong Wan 人参养荣丸				
Ze Lan (Hebra Lycopi) 泽兰	Root the Spirit *	Trypsin, Amylase, Pepsin.	The herbs, especially Di Yu, Wu Bei Zi and the patent medicines containing these herbs, restrict the proper function of the drugs.	Reduces therapeutic effect.	10, 13, 15.
Zhi Qiao (Fructus Aurantii) 枳壳	Run Chang Wan 润肠丸				
Zhi Shi (Fructus Aurantii Immaturus) 枳实	San Huang Shi Gao Tang 三黄石膏汤				
	Sang Ju Yin 桑菊饮				
	Sang Ju Gan Mao Pian 桑菊感冒片				
	Sha Shen Mai Dong Tang 沙参麦冬汤				
	Sheng Mai San 生脉散				
	Shi Chuan Da Bu Tang 十全大补汤				
	Si Ni San 四逆散				
	Si Wu Tang 四物汤				
	Stir Field of Elixir				
	Strengthen the Root				

* The samples do not have Chinese names

Table 7.3 (*Continued*)

Herbs	*Chinese Medicines*				
	Medicines	*Orthodox Drugs*	*Reasons*	*Results*	*Ref.*
	Tong Bi Wan 通痹丸				
	Wen Dan Tang 温胆汤				
	Wu Ji Bai Feng Wan 乌鸡白凤丸				
	Xiang Sha Yang Wei Tang 香砂养胃汤				
	Xiao Qing Long Tang 小青龙汤				
	Xiao Yao Wan 逍遥丸				
	Xue Fu Zhu Yu Tang 血府逐瘀汤				
	Yin Chen Tang 茵陈汤				
	You Gui Wan 右归丸				
	Yue Ju Wan 越鞠丸				
	Zhi Bo Di Huang Wan 知柏地黄丸				

Table 7.4 Interaction between Chinese Medicines containing Alkaloid and Orthodox Drugs (Ref. 5, 16, 17, 22, 23, 24)

Chinese Medicines		Orthodox Drugs	Reasons	Results	Ref.
Herbs	**Ready-made Medicines**				
Bai Bian Dou (Semen Lablab Album) 白扁豆	Ba Zhen Wan 八珍丸	Potassium Iodide, Sodium Iodide.	When the drugs are taken and mixed with gastric juices, iodite will be freed, but iodine and alkaloid will form precipitation.	Reduce absorption and therapeutic effect.	
Bai Bu (Radix Stemonae) 百部	Bai Du San 败毒散				
Bai He (Bulbus Lilii) 百合	Break into a Smile *				
Bai Xian Pi (Cortex Dictamni) 白鲜皮	Ban Xia Bai Zhu Tiar Ma Tang 半夏白术天麻汤				
Ban Xia (Rhizoma Pinelliae) 半夏	Ban Xia Hou Po Tang 半夏厚朴汤				
Ban Zhi Lian (Herba Scutellariae Barbata) 半枝莲	Ban Xia Xie Xin Tang 半夏泻心汤				
Bing Lang (Semen Arecae) 槟榔	Bao He Wan 保和丸	Sodium Bicarbonate.	The drugs affects the degree of dissociation of alkaloid.		
Cang Er Zi (Fructus Xanthii) 苍耳子	Bend Bamboo				
Chong Lou (Rhizoma Paridis) 重楼	Bi Xue Shen Shi Tang 萆薢渗湿汤				
Chuan Bei Mu (Bulbus Fritillariae Cirrhosae) 川贝母	Bi Yan Pian 鼻炎丸				
Chuan Xiong (Rhizoma Chuanxiong) 川芎	Brighten the Eyes	Bismuth Subcarbonate, Ferrous Sulfate,	The drugs are of metallic salts which will produce precipitation when taken with alkaloid.		
	Brocade Sinews *				
Da Fu Pi (Pericarpium Arecae) 大腹皮	Bu Zhong Yi Qi Wan 补中益气丸	Ferri Ammoni Cirtras,			
Da Ji (Radix Cirsii Japonic) 大蓟	Chai Hu Shu Gan Tang 柴胡疏肝汤	Aluminium Hydroxide,			
Dang Shen (Radix Codonoposis) 党参	Chemo Support	Magnesium Sulfate.			
Di Gu Pi (Cortex Lycii) 地骨皮	Chuan Bei Pi Pa Gao 川贝枇杷膏				
Da Huang (Radix Rehmanniae) 大黄	Chuan Xiong Che Tiao San 川芎茶调散				
Fu Zi (Radix Aconitilateralis Preparata) 附子	Clear Lustre				
	Clear the Soul *				
Gou Teng (Ramulus Uncariae Cum Uncis) 钩藤	Da Bu Yuan Jian 大补元煎				
	Da Chai Hu Tang 大柴胡汤				
Gua Lou (Fructus Trichosanthis) 瓜蒌	Da Qing Long Tang 大青龙汤				
Huai Jiao (Fructus Sophorae) 槐角	Du Huo Ji Sheng Tang 独活寄生汤				
Huang Bo (Cortex Phellodendri) 黄柏	Er Chen Wan 二陈丸				
Huang Jing (Rhizoma Polygonati) 黄精	Er Ming Zuo Ci Wan 耳鸣左慈丸				
Huang Lian (Rhizoma Coptidis) 黄连					

* The samples do not have Chinese names

Table 7.4 (Continued)

Herbs	Chinese Medicines – Ready-made Medicines		Orthodox Drugs	Reasons	Result	Ref.
Huang Qi (Radix Astragali) 黄芪	Fang Feng Tong Sheng San	防风通圣散				
Ji Li (Fructus Tribuli) 蒺藜	Freeing the Moon	*				
Jin Qian Cao (Herba Lysimachiae) 金钱草	Ge Xia Zhu Yu Tang	膈下逐瘀汤				
Ling Zhi (Ganoderma Lucidum Seu) 灵芝	Glorious Sea					
Long Kui (Solanom Nigrom) 龙葵	Gui Pi Wan	归脾丸				
Ma Chi Xian (Herba Portulacae) 马齿苋	Huang Qi Jian Zhong Tang	黄芪建中汤				
Ma Huang (Herba Ephedrae) 麻黄	Huo Xiang Zheng Qi Wan	藿香正气丸				
Ma Ren (Fructus Cannabis) 麻仁	Jade Spring	*				
Niu Xi (Radix Achyranthis Bidentata) 牛膝	Jin Suo Gu Jing Wan	金锁固精丸				
Shan Yao (Rhizoma Dioscoreae) 山药	Jing Fang Bai Du San	荆防败毒散				
Shen Jin Cao (Herba Lycopodii) 伸筋草	Jiu Wei Qiang Huo Wan	九味羌活丸				
Sheng Ma (Rhizoma Cimicifugae) 升麻	Liu Wei Di Huang Wan	六味地黄丸				
Tu Fu Ling (Rhozima Smilacis Glabrae) 土茯苓	Long Dan Xie Gan Tang	龙胆泻肝汤				
Wang Bu Liu Xing (Semen Vaccariae) 王不留行	Ma Huang Tang	麻黄汤				
Wu Jia Pi (Cortex Acanthopanacis) 五加皮	Ma Xing Shi Gan Tang	麻杏石甘汤				
Wu Zhu Yu (Fructus Evodiae) 吴茱萸	Ma Xing Yi Gan Tang	麻杏薏甘汤				
Xi Xian Cao (Herba Siegesbeckiae) 豨莶草	Ma Zi Ren Wan	麻子仁丸				
Xia Ku Cao (Spica Prunellae) 夏枯草	Ming Mu Di Huang Wan	明目地黄丸				
Xian Mao (Rhizoma Curculiginis) 仙茅	Open the Heart					
Xiao Ji (Herba Cirsii) 小蓟	Qi Ju Di Huang Wan	杞菊地黄丸				
Xu Duan (Radix Dipsaci) 续断	Qing Qi Hua Tan Wan	清气化痰丸				
Xuan Fu Hua (Flos Inulae) 旋覆花	Qing Wei San	清胃散				
Xuan Shen (Radix Scrophulariae) 玄参	Radio Support	*				
Yuan Hu (Rhizoma Corydalis) 元胡	Red Stirring	*				
Yi Mu Cao (Herba Leonuti) 益母草	Release Constraint					
Yu Zhu (Rhizoma Polygonati Odorati) 玉竹	Ren Shen Yang Rong Wan	人参养荣丸				
Ze Xie (Rhizoma Alismatis) 泽泻						

* The samples do not have Chinese names

Table 7.4 (Continued)

Herbs	Chinese Medicines		Orthodox Drugs	Reasons	Results	Ref.
		Ready-made Medicines				
Zhe Bei Mu (Bulbus Fritillariae Thunbergii)	浙贝母	Run Chang Wan 润肠丸				
Zi Hua Di Ding (Herba Violae)	紫花地丁	San Huang Shi Gao Tang 三黄石膏汤				
		Sha Shen Mai Dong Tang 沙参麦冬汤				
		Shi Quan Da Bu Wan 十全大补汤				
		Si Jun Zi Tang 四君子汤				
		Si Miao Yong An Tang 四妙勇安汤				
		Si Wu Tang 四物汤				
		Stir Field of Elixir *				
		Strengthen the Root *				
		Tong Bi Wan 通痹丸				
		Wen Dan Tang 温胆汤				
		Wu Ling San 五苓散				
		Wu Mei Wan 乌梅丸				
		Wu Ji Bai Feng Wan 乌鸡白凤丸				
		Xiang Sha Liu Jun Zi Wan 香砂六君子丸				
		Xiang Sha Yang Wei Tang 香砂养胃汤				
		Xiao Chai Hu Targ 小柴胡汤				
		Xiao Qing Long Tang 小青龙汤				
		Xue Fu Zhu Yu Tang 血府逐瘀汤				
		Yin Chen Wu Ling San 茵陈五苓散				
		You Gui Wan 右归丸				
		Yu Nu Jian 玉女煎				
		Yue Ju Wan 越鞠丸				
		Zhi Bo Di Huang Wan 知柏地黄丸				
		Zhu Ling Tang 猪苓汤				
		Zuo Gui Wan 左归丸				
		Zuo Jin Wan 左金丸				

* The samples do not have Chinese names

Table 7.5 Interaction between Chinese Medicines containing Quercetin and Orthodox Drugs (Ref. 5, 16, 17, 22, 23, 24)

Chinese Medicines		Orthodox Drugs	Reasons	Results	Ref.
Herbs	Ready-made Medicines				
Chai Hu (Radix Bupleuri) 柴胡	Bai Du San 败毒散	Calcium Gluconate,	Quercetin	Causes	6, 9, 10,
Ding Xiang (Flos Caryophylli) 丁香	Break into a Smile *	Calcium Carbonate,	consists of	difficulty in	25 (P290–294)
Hai Feng Teng (Caulis Piperis Kadsurae) 海风藤	Ban Xia Xie Xin Tang 半夏泻心汤	Calcium Lactate,	Phenol-Hydroxy,	absorption.	
	Bao He Wan 保和丸	Aluminium Hydroxide,	5-OH and		
He Huan Pi (Cortex Albizziae) 合欢皮	Bend Bamboo	Magnesium Sulphate,	4-Keto which		
Huai Hua (Flos Sophorae) 槐花	Bi Xue Shen Shi Tang 萆薢渗湿汤	Ferrous Sulphate,	will create		
Huai Jiao (Fructus Sophorae) 槐角	Bi Yan Pian 鼻炎片	Bismuth Subcarbonate.	precipitation		
Huang Bo (Cortex Phellodendri) 黄柏	Brocade Sinews		when taken		
Huang Lian (Rhizoma Coptidis) 黄连	Bu Zhong Yi Qi Wan 补中益气丸		with the drugs.		
Hu Zhang (Rhizoma Polygoni Cuspidati) 虎杖	Chai Ge Jie Ji Tang 柴葛解肌汤				
	Chai Hu Shu Gan Tang 柴胡疏肝汤				
Mei Gui Hua (Flos Rosae Rugosae) 玫瑰花	Clear the Soul *				
Mu Gua (Fructus Chaenomelis) 木瓜	Da Chai Hu Tang 大柴胡汤				
San Qi (Radix Notoginseng) 三七	Dang Gui Si Ni Tang 当归四逆汤				
Sang Ji Sheng (Herba Taxilli) 桑寄生	Du Huo Ji Sheng Tang 独活寄生汤				
Sang Ye (Folium Mori) 桑叶	Er Ming Zuo Ci Wan 耳鸣左慈丸				
Shan Zha (Fructus Crataegi) 山楂	Freeing the Moon *				
Yu Xing Cao (Herba Houttuyniae) 鱼腥草	Ge Xia Zhu Yu Tang 膈下逐瘀汤				
Yu Zhu (Radix Polygalae) 玉竹	Jade Spring *				

* The samples do not have Chinese names

Table 7.5 (Continued)

Herbs	Chinese Medicines		Orthodox Drugs	Reasons	Results	Ref.
	Ready-made Medicines					
Zi Yuan (Radix Asteris)	紫苑	Jing Fang Bai Du San	荆防败毒散				
		Liu Wei Di Huang Wan	六味地黄丸				
		Long Dan Xie Gan Tang	龙胆泻肝汤				
		Open the Heart	*				
		Qing Qi Hua Tan Wan	清气化痰丸				
		Qing Wei San	清胃散				
		Red Stirring	*				
		San Huang Shi Gac Tang	三黄石膏汤				
		Sang Ju Yin	桑菊饮				
		Sang Ju Gan Mao Pian	桑菊感冒片				
		Sha Shen Mai Dong Tang	沙参麦冬汤				
		Si Ni San	四逆散				
		Stir Field of Elixir	*				
		Tong Bi Wan	通鼻丸				
		Wu Ji Bai Feng Wan	乌鸡白凤丸				
		Wu Mei Wan	乌梅丸				
		Xiao Chai Hu Tang	小柴胡汤				
		Xiao Yao Wan	逍遥丸				
		Xue Fu Zhu Yu Tang	血府逐瘀汤				
		Zhi Bo Di Huang Wan	知柏地黄丸				
		Zuo Jin Wan	左金丸				

* The samples do not have Chinese names

Table 7.6 Interaction between Chinese Medicines containing Acid and Orthodox Drugs (Ref. 5, 16, 17, 22, 23, 24)

Herbs	Ready-made Medicines		Orthodox Drugs	Reasons	Results	Ref.
Ba Ji Tian (Radix Morindae Officinalis) 巴戟天	Bai Du San	败毒散	Sodium Bicarbonate, Aluminium Hydroxide	The drugs are alkali which neutralize acid.	The effect of both medicines and drugs are lost.	6, 10, 13
Che Qian Cao (Herba Plantaginis) 车前草	Bao He Wan	保和丸				
Che Qian Zi (Semen Plantaginis) 车前子	Bi Yan Pian	鼻炎片	Aminoglycosides (Kanamycin, Amikacin, *Dihydros-Treptomycin,* Framycetin, Neomycin, Gentamicin, Paromomycin, Sisomicin, Stretomycin, Tobramycin)	The acid decreases the antibiotic effect of the drugs.	Reduces therapeutic effect.	6, 8, 9, 13, 14
He Zi (Fructus Chebulate) 诃子	Brighten the Eyes	*				
Ma Chi Xian (Herba Portulacae) 马齿苋	Bu Zhong Yi Qi Wan	补中益气丸				
Mao Gen (Rhizoma Imperatae) 茅根	Chemo Support	*				
Mu Gua (Fructus Chaenomelis) 木瓜	Chuan Bei Pi Pa Gao	川贝枇杷膏				
Nu Zhen Zi (Fructus Ligustri Lucidi) 女贞子	Da Bu Yuan Jian	大补元煎				
Shan Zha (Fructus Cartaegi) 山楂	Da Chai Hu Tang	大柴胡汤				
Shan Zhu Yu (Fructus Corni) 山茱萸	Da Cheng Qi Tang	大承气汤				
Sheng Ma (Rhizoma Cimicitugae) 升麻	Er Ming Zuo Ci Wan	耳鸣左慈丸				
Wu Mei (Fructus Mume) 乌梅	Fang Feng Tong Sheng San	防风通圣散	*Reserpin, caffein,* opium, Scopolamin, Berbamin	The chemical structures of the drugs change when encountering an acid, resulting in decrease in reabsorption of renal tabules and profuse excretion of the drugs in the urine.	Reduces the effect of the drugs.	6
Wu Wei Zi (Fructus Schisandrae) 五味子	Long Dan Xie Gan Tang	龙胆泻肝汤				
Zhi Qiao (Fructus Aurantii) 枳壳	Ming Mu Di Huang Wan	明目地黄丸				
Zhi Shi (Fructus Aurantii Immaturus) 枳实	Qi Ju Di Huang Wan	杞菊地黄丸				
	Qing Qi Hua Tan Wan	清气化痰丸				
	Radio Support	*				
	Sheng Mai San	生脉散				
	Wu Mei Wan	乌梅丸				
	Xiao Qing Long Tang	小青龙汤				
	Zhi Bo Di Huang Wan	知柏地黄丸				

* The samples do not have Chinese names

Table 7.6 (Continued)

Chinese Medicines					
Herbs	Ready-made Medicines	Orthodox Drugs	Reasons	Results	Ref.
		Erythromycine	The chemical structure of the drug is destroyed and the antibacterial action is lost.	Loses therapeutic effect.	6, 14, 15
		Sulphasalazine, Sulphonamides (Sulphadiazine, Sulphadimethoxine, Sulphadimdine, Sulphafurazole, Sulphamerazine, Sulphamethizole, Sulphamethoxypyridazine, Sulphaphenazole, Sulphasomidine, Sulphathiazole)	Acid occurs in the urine resulting in decreasing the solubility of the drugs.	Causes the production of Crystalluria and Hematuria.	13, 14

Table 7.7 Interaction between Chinese Medicines containing Akali and Orthodox Drugs (Ref. 5, 16, 17, 25)

Chinese Medicines			Orthodox Drugs	Reasons	Results	Ref.
Herbs		Ready-made Medicines				
Bai Xian Pi (Cortex Dictamni)	白鲜皮	Ming Mu Di Huang Tang 明目地黄汤	Tetracyclines (Tetracycline, Rolitetracycline, Oxytetracycline, Aureomycicline, Doxycycline, Declomycine, Methacycline, Demellocycline, Minocycline) Penicillin G, Amoxicillin, Polymyxin, Furadantin.	The solubility of the drugs is decreased.	Reduces therapeutic effect.	6, 14
Bing Lang (Semen Arecae)	槟榔	Glorious Sea *				
Ku Shen (Radix Sophorae Flavescens)	苦参	Stir Field of Elixir *				
Peng Sha (Borax)	硼砂	Clear Lustre *				
Shi Jue Ming (Haliotis Diversicolor)	石决明					
Yuan Hu (Rhizoma Corydalis)	元胡					
			Aminoglycosides (Streptomycin, Kanamycin, Neomycin)	The concentration of the drugs in the brain tissue is increased.	Causes vestibulcochlear nerve poison.	6, 9
			Quinidine	The reabsorption at the kidney tubules is increased, resulting in retention of quinidine.	Causes quinidine intoxication.	6

* The samples do not have Chinese names

Table 7.8 Interaction between Chinese Medicines containing Potassium and Orthodox Drugs (Ref. 5, 7, 18, 23, 24, 25)

Chinese Medicines				Orthodox Drugs	Reasons	Results	Ref.
Herbs		Ready-made Medicines					
Bai Mao Gen (Rhizoma Imperatae)	白茅根	Ba Zhen Wan	八珍丸	Antisterone	The drugs belong	Develops	7,
Bai Shao (Radix Paeoniae Alba)	白芍	Bai Du San	败毒散	Spironolactone	to Potassium	Hyperkalaemia.	21 (P453)
Ban Lan Gen (Radix Isatidis)	板蓝根	Bai Hu Tang	白虎汤	Triamterene	Sparing Diuretics		25 (P327-
Bian Xu (Hweba Polygomi Avicularis)	萹蓄	Break into a Smile	*	Amiloride	and they cause		330)
Chai Hu (Radix Bupleuri)	柴胡	Ban Xia Bai Zhu Tian Ma Tang	半夏白术天麻汤		retention of		
Chen Pi (Pericarpium Citrireticulatae)	陈皮				potassium. The		
Chi Shao (Radix Paeonia Rubra)	赤芍	Ban Xia Hou Po Tang	半夏厚朴汤		Chinese medicines		
Chuan Xiong (Rhizoma Chuanxiong)	川芎	Ban Xia Xie Xin Tang	半夏泻心汤		also contain		
Dai Fu Pi (Pericarpium Arecae)	大腹皮	Bao He Wan	保和丸		potassium.		
Da Huang (Radix Et Rhixoma Rhei)	大黄	Bend Bamboo	*		Excessive		
Dang Pi (Cortex Moutan)	丹皮	Bi Xie Fen Qing Yin	萆薢分清饮		potassium will		
Dan Shen (Radix Salviae Miltiorrhizae)	丹参	Bi Xie Shen Shi Tang	萆薢渗湿汤		result when both		
Dan Zhu Ye (Herba Lophathebi)	淡竹叶	Bi Yan Pian	鼻炎丸		are taken together.		
Dang Gui (Radix Angelica Sinensis)	当归	Brighten the Eyes	*				
Dang Shen (Radix Codonopsis)	党参	Brocade Sinews	*				
Fu Ling (Poria)	茯苓	Bu Zhong Yi Qi Wan	补中益气丸				
Fu Ping (Spirodela Polyrrhiza)	浮萍	Chi Feng Zhen Zhu An Chuang Wan	彩凤珍珠暗疮丸				
Gan Cao (Radix Glycyrrhizae)	甘草	Chai Ge Jie Ji Tang	柴葛解肌汤				
Gou Teng (Ramulus Uncariae Cum Uncis)	钩藤	Chai Hu Shu Gan Tang	柴胡疏肝汤				
Hai Zao (Sargassum)	海藻	Chemo Support	*				
Han Lian Cao (Eclipth Prostrata)	旱莲草	Chuan Bei Pi Pa Gao	川贝枇杷膏				
Hong Hua (Flos Carthami)	红花	Chuan Xiong Cha Tiao San	川芎茶调散				
Hou Po (Cortex Magnoliae Officinalis)	厚朴	Clear Lustre	*				
		Clear the Soul	*				
Huang Jing (Rhizoma Polygonati)	黄精	Da Bu Yuan Jian	大补元煎				
Huang Lian (Rhizoma Coptidis)	黄连	Da Chai Hu Tang	大柴胡汤				
Huang Qi (Radix Astragali)	黄芪	Da Cheng Qi Tang	大承气汤				
		Da Qing Long Tang	大青龙汤				

* The samples do not have Chinese names

Table 7.8 *(Continued)*

	Chinese Medicines				
Herbs	Ready-made Medicines	Orthodox Drugs	Reasons	Results	Ref.
Huang Qin (Radix Scutellariae) 黄芩	Dan Shen Pian 丹参片				
Jin Qian Cao (Herba Lysimachiae) 金钱草	Dang Gui Si Ni Tang 当归四逆汤				
Jin Yin Hua (Flos Lonicerae) 金银花	Dao Chi San 导赤散				
Ku Shen (Radix Sophorae Flavescens) 苦参	Du Huo Ji Sheng Tang 独活寄生汤				
Ku Xing Ren (Semen Armaniacae Amarum) 苦杏仁	Er Chen Wan 二陈丸				
Kun Bu (Thallus Laminariae) 昆布	Er Ming Zuo Ci Wan 耳鸣左慈丸				
Lian Qiao (Fructus Forsythiae) 连翘	Fang Feng Tong Shen San 防风通圣散				
Long Gu (Os Draconis) 龙骨	Freeing the Moon *				
Ma Chi Xian (Herba Portulacae) 马齿苋	Gan Mao Lin 感冒灵				
Ma Huang (Herba Ephedrae) 麻黄	Ge Xie Zhu Yu Tang 膈下逐瘀汤				
Mu Tong (Caulis Celmatidis Armandii) 木通	Glorious Sea *				
Niu Bang Zi (Fructus Arctii) 牛蒡子	Gui Pi Wan 归脾丸				
Niu Xi (Radix Achyranthis Bidentata) 牛膝	Gui Zhi Tang 桂枝汤				
	Huang Qi Jian Zhong Tang 黄芪建中汤				
Nu Zhen Zi (Fructus Ligustrilucidi) 女贞子	Huo Xiang Zheng Qi Wan 藿香正气丸				
Pu Gong Ying (Herba Taraxaci) 蒲公英	Jade Spring *				
Pu Huang (Pollen Typhae) 蒲黄	Jing Fang Bai Du San 荆防败毒散				
Qi Zi (Fructus Lycii) 杞子	Jiu Wei Qiang Huo Wan 九味羌活丸				
Qing Hao (Herba Artemisia Annuae) 青蒿	Li Zhong Wan 理中丸				
Rou Gui (Cortex Cinnamomi) 肉桂	Liu Wei Di Huang Wan 六味地黄丸				
Sang Ji Sheng (Herba Taxilli) 桑寄生	Liu Yi San 六一散				
Sang Piao Xiao (Ootheca Mantidis) 桑螵蛸	Long Dan Xie Gan Tang 龙胆泻肝汤				
Sang Shen (Fructus Mori) 桑椹	Ma Huang Tang 麻黄汤				
Shan Yao (Rixoma Dioscoreae) 山药	Ma Xing Shi Gan Tang 麻杏石甘汤				
She Jin Cao (Herba Lycopodii) 伸筋草	Ma Xing Yi Gan Tang 麻杏薏甘汤				
Sheng Di Huang (Rehmannia Glutinosa) 生地黄	Ma Zi Ren Wan 麻子仁汤				
	Ming Mu Di Huang Wan 明目地黄丸				

* The samples do not have Chinese names

Table 7.8 (Continued)

	Chinese Medicines			Orthodox Drugs	Reasons	Results	Ref.
Herbs		Ready-made Medicines					
Tai Zi Shen (Radix Pseudostellariae)	太子参	Open the Heart					
		Ping Wei San	平胃散	*			
Tao Ren (Semen Persicae)	桃仁	Qi Ju Di Huang Wan	杞菊地黄丸				
Tian Hua Fen (Radix Trichosanthis)	天花粉	Qing Qi Hua Tan Wan	清气化痰丸				
Tu Fu Ling (Rhizoma Smilacisglabrae)	土茯苓	Qing Wei San	清胃散	*			
		Red Stirring					
Tu Si Zi (Semen Cuscutae)	兔丝子	Release Constraint		*			
Wu Wei Zi (Fructus Schisandrae)	五味子	Ren Shen Yang Rong Wan	人参养荣丸				
Xi Xian Cao (Herba Siegesbeckiae)	豨莶草	Root the Spirit		*			
Xia Ku Cao (Spica Prunellae)	夏枯草	Run Chang Wan	润肠丸				
Xiao Ji (Herba Cirsii)	小蓟	San Huang Shi Gao Tang	三黄石膏汤				
Xu Duan (Radix Dipsaci)	铁断	Sang Ju Gan Mao Pian	桑菊感冒片				
Xuan Shen (Radix Scophulariae)	玄参	Sang Ju Yin	桑菊饮				
Yi Mu Cao (Herba Leonuti)	益母草	Sha Shen Mai Dong Tang	沙参麦冬汤				
Yi Ren (Seman Coicis)	薏仁						
Yi Zhi Ren (Fructus Alpiniae Oxyphyllae)	益智仁	Shi Chuan Da Bu Tang	十全大补汤				
		Si Miao Yong An Tang	四妙勇安汤				
Yin Chen (Herba Artemisiae Scopariae)	茵陈	Si Ni San	四逆散				
		Si Jun Zi Tang	四君子汤				
Yin Yang Huo (Herba Epimedii)	淫羊藿	Si Wu Tang	四物汤				
Yu Jin (Darix Curcumae)	郁金	Stir Field of Elixir		*			
Yu Xing Cao (Herba Houttuyniae)	鱼腥草	Strengthen the Root					
Ze Xie (Rhizoma Alismatis)	泽泻	Tong Bi Wan	通鼻丸				
Zhi Mu (Rhizoma Anemarrhenae)	知母	Wen Dan Tang	温胆汤				
Zhi Zi (Fructus Gardeniae)	栀子	Wen Jing Tang	温经汤				
Zhu Ru (Caulis Bambusaein Taemam)	竹茹	Wu Ji Bai Feng Wan	乌鸡白凤丸				
		Wu Ling San	五苓散				

* The samples do not have Chinese names

Table 7.8 (Continued)

| Herbs | Chinese Medicines | | | | |
	Ready-made Medicines	Orthodox Drugs	Reasons	Results	Ref.
	Wu Mei Wan 乌梅丸				
	Xiang Sha Liu Jun Zi Wan 香砂六君子丸				
	Xiang Sha Yang Wei Tang 香砂养胃汤				
	Xiao Chai Hu Tang 小柴胡汤				
	Xiao Qing Long Tang 小青龙汤				
	Xiao Yao Wan 逍遥丸				
	Xue Fu Zhu Yu Tang 血府逐瘀汤				
	Yin Chen Tang 茵陈汤				
	Yin Chen Wu Ling San 茵陈五苓散				
	Yin Qiao Jie Du Pian 银翘解毒片				
	You Gui Yin 右归饮				
	Yu Nu Jian 玉女煎				
	Yue Ju Wan 越鞠丸				
	Zhi Bo Di Huang Wan 知柏地黄丸				
	Zhu Ling Tang 猪苓汤				
	Zuo Gui Wan 左归丸				
	Zuo Jin Wan 左金丸				

Table 7.9 Interaction between Chinese Medicines containing Amylase and Orthodox Drugs (Ref. 5, 7, 17, 23, 24, 25)

Chinese Medicines			Orthodox Drugs	Reasons	Results	Ref.
Herbs		Ready-made Medicines				
Dan Dou Chi (Semen Sojae Preparatum)	淡豆豉	Bao He Wan	保和丸	Tetracyclines (Tetracycline, Rolitetracycline, Oxytetracycline, Aureomycicline, Doxycycline, Declomycine, Minocycline, Methacycline, Demeclocycline)	These drugs are not compatible with Amylase. They destroy activities of Amylase.	Reduces therapeutic effect.	6, 8, 14
Gu Ya (Fructus Oryzae Sativae Germinatus)	谷芽	Brighten the Eyes	*				
Mai Ya (Fructus Hordei Germinatus)	麦芽	Chemo Support	*				
Shan Yao (Rhizoma Dioscoreae)	山药	Da Bu Yuan Jian	大补元煎				
Shen Qu (Massa Fermentata Medicalis)	神曲	Er Ming Zuo Ci Wan	耳鸣左慈丸				
Tian Nan Xing (Rhizoma Arisaematis)	天南星	Glorious Sea	*				
Tu Si Zi (Semen Cuscutae)	菟丝子	Jade Spring	*				
		Jing Fang Bai Du San	荆防败毒散				
		Liu Wei Di Huang Wan	六味地黄丸				
		Ming Mu Di Huang Wan	明目地黄丸				
		Qi Ju Di Huang Wan	杞菊地黄丸				
		Qing Qi Hua Tan Wan	清气化痰丸				
		Release Constraint	*	Sulphonamides (Sulphadiazine, Sulphadimethoxine, Sulphadimdine, Sulphafurazole, Sulphamerazine, Sulphamethizole, Sulphamethoxypyridazine, Sulphamethpyrazine, Sulphaphenazole, Sulphasomidine, Sulphathiazole)			
		Root the Spirit	*				
		Strengthen the Root	*				
		Wu Ji Bai Feng Wan	乌鸡白凤丸				
		Yin Qiao Jie Du Pian	银翘解毒片				
		You Gui Wan	右归丸				
		Yue Ju Wan	越鞠丸				
		Zhi Bo Di Huang Wan	知柏地黄丸				
		Zuo Gui Wan	左归丸				
				Aspirin			

* The samples do not have Chinese names

Table 7.10 Interaction between Chinese Medicines containing Glycoside and Orthodox Drugs (Ref. 5, 11, 18, 23, 24, 25)

Herbs		Ready-made Medicines		Orthodox Drugs	Reasons	Results	Ref.
	Chinese Medicines						
Bai Guo (Semen Ginkgo)	白果	Ba Zhen Wan	八珍丸	Vitamin C	These group of	Reduces	6
Bai Jiang Cao (Herba Patriniae)	败酱草	Bai Du San	败毒散	Nicotinic Acid,	Chinese medicines	therapeutic	
Bai Shao (Radix Paeoniae Alba)	白芍	Break into a Smile	*	Glutamic Acid,	are not compatible	effect.	
Bai Tou Weng (Radix Pulsatillae)	白头翁	Ban Xia Bai Zhu Tian Ma Tang	半夏白术天麻汤	Hydrochloric Acid.	with acidic drugs		
Bai Zi Ren (Semen Platycladi)	柏子仁				which destroy the		
Bai Xian Pi (Cortex Dictamni)	白鲜皮	Ban Xia Hou Po Tang	半夏厚朴汤		Glycoside activities		
Ban Lan Gen (Radix Isatidis)	板蓝根	Ban Xia Xie Xin Tang	半夏泻心汤				
Ban Xia (Rhizoma Pinelliae)	半夏	Bao He Wan	保和丸				
Bi Xie (Rhizoma Dioscoreae)	萆薢	Bend Bamboo	*				
Cang Er Zi (Fructus Xan Thii)	苍耳子	Bi Xie Fen Qing Yin	萆薢分清饮				
Chai Hu (Radix Bupleuri)	柴胡	Bix Xie Shen Shi Tang	萆薢渗湿汤				
Che Qian Zi (Semen Plantaginis)	车前子	Bi Yan Pian	鼻炎片				
Chi Shao (Radix Paeonia Rubra)	赤芍	Brighten the Eyes	*				
Chong Lou (Rhizoma Paridis)	重楼	Brocade Sinews	*				
Da Huang (Radix Et Rhizoma Rhei)	大黄	Bu Zhong Yi Qi Wan	补中益气丸				
Da Ji (Radix Crsii Japonici)	大蓟	Chemo Support	*				
Da Qing Ye (Folium Isatidis)	大青叶	Chai Ge Jie Ji Tang	柴葛解肌汤				
Dan Pi (Cortex Moutan)	丹皮	Chi Feng Zhen Zhu An Chuang Wan	彩凤珍珠暗疮丸				
Dang Shen (Radix Codonopsis)	党参						
Di Fu Zi (Fructus Kochiae)	地肤子	Chuan Bei Pi Pa Gao	川贝枇杷膏				
Di Yu (Radix Sanguisorbae)	地榆	Chuan Xiong Cha Tiao San	川芎茶调散				
Fan Xie Ye (Folium Sennae)	番泻叶						
Fang Feng (Radix Saposhnikoviae)	防风	Clear the Soul	*				
Gua Lou (Fructus Trichosanthis)	瓜蒌	Clear Lustre					
Gu Sui Bu (Rhizoma Drynariae)	骨碎补	Da Bu Yuan Jian	大补元煎				
He Huan Pi (Cortex Albizziae)	合欢皮	Da Chai Hu Tang	大柴胡汤				
Hong Hua (Flos Carthami)	红花	Da Cheng Qi Tang	大承气汤				
Huai Hua (Flos Sophorae)	槐花	Dang Gui Si Ni Tang	当归四逆汤				
Huai Jiao (Fructus Sophorae)	槐角	Du Huo Ji Sheng Tang	独活寄生汤				
Huang Qin (Radix Scutellariae)	黄芩	Er Chen Wan	二陈丸				

* The samples do not have Chinese names

Table 7.10 *(Continued)*

	Chinese Medicines		Orthodox Drugs	Reasons	Results	Ref.
Herbs	**Ready-made Medicines**					
Ji Li (Fructus Tribuli) 蒺藜	Er Ming Zuo Ci Wan	耳鸣左慈丸				
Jie Geng (Radix Platycodi) 桔梗	Fang Feng Tong Sheng San	防风通圣散				
Jin Qian Cao (Herba Lysimachiae) 金钱草	Freeing the Moon	*				
Jin Yin Hua (Flos Lonicerae) 金银花	Gan Mao Lin	感冒灵				
Kuan Dong Hua (Flos Farfarae) 款冬花	Ge Xia Zhu Yu Tang	膈下逐瘀汤				
Ku Xing Ren (Semen Armeniacae Amarum) 苦杏仁	Glorious Sea					
Lian Qiao (Fructus Forsythiae) 连翘	Gui Pi Wan	归脾丸				
Long Dan Cao (Radix Gentiana) 龙胆草	Gui Zhi Tang	桂枝汤				
Ma Chi Xian (Herba Portulacae) 马齿苋	Huang Qi Jian Zhong Tang	黄芪建中汤				
Mai Dong (Radix Ophiopogonis) 麦冬	Huo Xiang Zhen Qi Wan	藿香正气丸				
Mu Gua (Fructus Chaenomelis) 木瓜	Jade Spring	*				
Nan Sha Shen (Radix Adenophorae) 南沙参	Jing Fang Bai Du San	荆防败毒散				
Niu Bang Zi (Fructus Arctii) 牛蒡子	Jiu Wei Qiang Huo Wan	九味羌活丸				
Niu Xi (Radix Cyathulae) 牛膝	Li Zhong Wan	理中丸				
Nu Zhen Zi (Fructus Ligustrilucidi) 女贞子	Liu Wei Di Huang Wan	六味地黄丸				
Pi Pa Ye (Folium Eriobotryae) 枇杷叶	Long Dan Xie Gan Tang	龙胆泻肝汤				
Pu Gong Ying (Herba Taraxaci) 清公英	Ma Zi Ren Wan	麻子仁丸				
Qin Pi (Cortex Traxini) 秦皮	Ming Mu Di Huang Wan	明目地黄丸				
Qu Mai (Herba Dianthi) 瞿麦	Open the Heart					
Ren Dong Teng (Caulis Lonicerae) 忍冬藤	Qi Ju Di Huang Wan	杞菊地黄丸				
Ren Shen (Radix Ginseng) 人参	Qing Qi Hua Tan Wan	清气化痰丸				
San Qi (Radix Notoginseng) 三七	Qing Wei San	清胃散				
Sang Ji Sheng (Herba Taxilli) 桑寄生	Radio Support	*				
Sheng Ma (Rhizoma Cimicifugae) 升麻	Red Stirring	*				
Shan Yao (Rhizoma Dioscoreae) 山药	Release Constraint	*				
Shan Zha (Fructus Crataegi) 山楂	Ren Shen Yang Rong Wan	人参养荣丸				
Shan Zhu Yu (Fructus Cormi) 山茱萸	Root the Spirit					
Tai Zi Shen (Radix Pseudostellariaf) 太子参	Run Chang Wan	润肠丸				
Tao Ren (Semen Persicae) 桃仁	San Huang Shi Gac Tang	三黄石膏汤				
Tian Hua Fen (Radix Trichosanthis) 天花粉						

* The samples do not have Chinese names

Table 7.10 (Continued)

Herbs	Chinese Medicines		Orthodox Drugs	Reasons	Results	Ref.
	Ready-made Medicines					
Tian Ma (Rhixoma Gastrodiae) 天麻	Sang Ju Yin	桑菊饮				
Tian Nan Xing (Rhizoma Arisaematis) 天南星	Sang Ju Gang Mao Pian	桑菊感冒片				
Tu Fu Ling (Rhizoma Smilacis Glabrae) 土茯苓	Sha Shen Mai Dong Tang	沙参麦冬汤				
	Sheng Mai San	生脉散				
Tu Si Zi (Semen Cuscutae) 菟丝子	Shi Quan Da Bu Wan	十全大补丸				
Wei Ling Xian (Herba Clematidis) 威灵仙	Si Jun Zi Tang	四君子汤				
Xi Yang Shen (Radix Panacis Quinquefolii) 西洋参	Si Miao Yong An Tang	四妙勇安汤				
	Si Ni San	四逆散				
Xian He Cao (Herba Agrimoniae) 仙鹤草	Si Wu Tang	四物汤				
Xiao Ji (Herba Cirsii) 小蓟	Stir Field of Elixir	*				
Xuan Shen (Radix Scrophulariae) 玄参	Strengthen the Root	*				
Yin Yang Huo (Herba Epimedii) 淫羊藿	Wen Dan Tang	温胆汤				
Yu Mi Xu (Stigma Maydis) 玉米须	Wu Ji Bai Feng Wan	乌鸡白凤丸				
Yu Xing Cao (Herba Houttuyniae) 鱼腥草	Wu Mei Wan	乌梅丸				
Yu Zhu (Rhizoma Polygonati Odorati) 玉竹	Xiang Sha Liu Jun Zi Wan	香砂六君子丸				
Yuan Zhi (Radix Polygalae) 远志	Xiang Sha Yang Wei Wan	香砂养胃丸				
Zhi Mu (Rhizoma Anemarrhenae) 知母	Xiao Chai Hu Tang	小柴胡汤				
Zhi Qiao (Fructus Aurantii) 枳壳	Xiao Qing Long Tang	小青龙汤				
Zhi Zi (Fructus Gardeniae) 栀子	Xiao Yao Wan	逍遥丸				
Zi Hua Di Ding (Herba Violae) 紫花地丁	Yin Chen Tang	茵陈汤				
Zi Yuan (Radix Asteris) 紫菀	Yin Qiao (Chiao) Jie Du Pian	银翘解毒片				
	You Gui Wan	右归丸				
	Yu Nu Jian	玉女煎				
	Yue Ju Wan	越鞠丸				
	Zhi Bo Di Huang Wan	知柏地黄丸				
	Zuo Gui Wan	左归丸				

* The samples do not have Chinese names

Table 7.11 Interaction between Chinese Medicines containing Cyanophoric Glycoside and Orthodox Drugs (Ref. 5, 16, 17, 23, 24, 25)

Chinese Medicines			Orthodox Drugs	Reasons	Results	Ref.
Herbs		Ready-made Medicines				
Bai Guo (Semen Ginko)	白果	Chuan Bei Pi Pa Gao	川贝枇杷膏	Codeine Phosphate	Hydrocyanic	Inhibits	6, 8, 14,
Ku Xing Ren (Semen Armeniacae)	苦杏仁	Da Qing Long Tang	大青龙汤	Morphine	acid is	respiratory	25 (P152)
Tao Ren (Semen Persicae)	桃仁	Ge Xia Zhu Yu Tang	膈下逐瘀汤	Pethidine	produced.	centre.	
		Ma Huang Tang	麻黄汤	Benzobarbiton			
		Ma Xing Shi Gan Tang	麻杏石甘汤				
		Ma Xing Yi Gan Tang	麻杏薏甘汤				
		Ma Zi Ren Wan	麻子仁丸				
		Run Chang Wan	润肠丸				
		Sang Ju Gan Mao Pian	桑菊感冒片				
		Sang Ju Yin	桑菊饮				
		Xue Fu Zhu Yu Tang	血府逐瘀汤				

Table 7.12 Interaction between Chinese Ready-made Medicines containing Chinese Herb Gan Cao (Radix Gycyrrhizae) & Orthodox Drugs

Chinese Ready-made Medicines		Orthodox Drugs	Reasons	Results	Ref.
Ba Zhen Wan	八珍丸	Quinine, Ephedrine, Atropine	Interaction will result in precipitation.	Reduces therapeutic effect.	6, 8
Bai Du San	敗毒散				
Break into a Smile					
Bai Hu Tang	白虎汤	Digitoxin, Digoxin	Gan Cao contains cortisone-like substances while Digitalis is a cardioactive steroid glycoside. If combined, intoxication will be caused.	Results in Digitalism.	6, 8
Bend Bamboo					
Bi Xie Fen Qing Yin	萆薢分清饮				
Bi Yan Pian	鼻炎片				
Brocade Sinews					
Chemo Support					
Chai Ge Jie Ji Tang	柴葛解肌汤				
Chai Hu Shu Gan Tang	柴胡疏肝汤	Insulin, Tolbutamide	Gan Cao contains cortisone-like substances which will increase blood sugar and defeat the action of the drugs	Blood sugar cannot be reduced effectively.	6, 8, 10 13, 15
Chuan Bei Pi Pa Gao	川贝枇杷膏				
Chuan Xiong Cha Tiao San	川芎茶调散				
Clear Lustre					
Clear the Soul					
Da Qing Long Tang	大青龙汤	Sodium Salicylate, Aspirin	Both the Chinese medicines and the drugs have similar action of being gastric irritant.	Increases Gastric ulceration.	6, 8, 10
Dang Gui Si Ni Tang	当归四逆汤				
Dao Chi San	导赤散				
Du Huo Ji Sheng Tang	独活寄生汤				
Er Chen Wan	二陈丸				
Fang Feng Tong Sheng San	防风通圣散	Hydrochlorothiazide, Acetazolamindum, Furosemide, Chlorthalidone	The use of these drugs can produce Hypokalemia and Gan Cao also has the same reaction.	Increases the risk of Hypokalemia.	6, 8
Freeing the Moon					
Ge Xia Zhu Yu Tang	膈下逐瘀汤				
Glorious Sea	*				
Gui Pi Wan	归脾丸				
Gui Zhi Tang	桂枝汤	Amphotericin	Both cause Potassium loss.	Causes heart failure.	14
Huang Qi Jian Zhong Tang	黄芪建中汤				
Huo Xiang Zheng Qi Wan	藿香正气丸	Isoniazid, Rifampicin	Gan Cao reduces the concurrent use of the drugs.	Spreads T.B.	14
Jade Spring	*				
Jing Fang Bai Du San	荆防败毒散				

* The samples do not have Chinese names

Table 7.12 (Continued)

Chinese Ready-made Medicines		Orthodox Drugs	Reasons	Results	Ref.
Jiu Wei Qiang Huo Wan	九味羌活丸	Erythromycin	When Gan Cao and the drugs are used together, absorption rate of the drugs will be reduced.	Reduces antibiotic effect.	14
Li Zhong Wan	理中丸	Chloramphenical,			
Liu Yi San	六一散	Tetracyclines			
Long Dan Xie Gan Tang	龙胆泻肝汤	(Tetracycline,			
Ma Huang Tang	麻黄汤	Rolitetracycline,			
Ma Xing Shi Gan Tang	麻杏石甘汤	Oxytetracycline,			
Ma Xing Yi Gan Tang	麻杏薏甘汤	Aureomycycline,			
Open the Heart	*	Doxycycline,			
Ping Wei San	平胃散	Declomycine,			
Radio Support	*	Minccycine,			
Red Stirring	*	Methacycline,			
Release Constraint	*	Demeclocycline)			
Ren Shen Yang Rong Wan	人参养荣丸				
Sang Ju Yin	桑菊饮				
Sha Shen Mai Dong Tang	沙参麦冬汤				
Si Jun Zi Tang	四君子汤				
Si Ni Tang	四逆汤				
Stir Field of Elixir	*				
Strengthen the Root	*				
Tong Bi Wan	通鼻丸				
Wen Dan Tang	温胆汤				
Wu Ji Bai Feng Wan	乌鸡白凤丸				
Xiang Sha Liu Jun Zi Wan	香砂六君子丸				
Xiang Sha Yang Wei Tang	香砂养胃汤				
Xiao Chai Hu Tang	小柴胡汤				
Xiao Yao Wan	逍遥丸				
Xiao Qing Long Tang	小青龙汤				
Xue Fu Zhu Yu Tang	血府逐瘀汤				
Yin Qiao Jie Du Pian	银翘解毒片				
You Gui Yin	右归饮				

* The samples do not have Chinese names

Table 7.13　Interaction between Chinese Ready-made Medicines containing Chinese Herb Ma Huang (Herba Ephedrae) & Orthodox Drugs

Chinese Ready-made Medicines	Orthodox Drugs	Reasons	Results	Ref.
Bi Yan Pian 鼻炎片 Da Qing Long Tang 大青龙汤 Fang Feng Tong Sheng San 防风通圣散 Ma Huang Tang 麻黄汤 Ma Xing Shi Gan Tang 麻杏石甘汤 Ma Xing Yi Gan Tang 麻杏薏甘汤 Xiao Qing Long Tang 小青龙汤	Digitalis (Digitoxin, Digoxin)	The effect of Digitalis is enhanced	Causes Cardiac Arrythmia	6, 8, 11
	Phenal Barbiturate	Both are Antagonizers	Antagonizes Sedative Effect	6, 11
	Adrenaline, Isoprenaline	Contraction of blood vessel wall is enhanced	Causes Hypertension	6, 8, 11
	Aminophylline	Blood pressure is increased	Causes Palpitation or Headaches	6, 8, 11
	Furazolidon, Phenelzine, Phenylamine, Isoniazid Isocarboxazid, Eutonyl, Procarbazine, Nialamide, Tolylhydrazine	Ma Huang releases Noradrenaline, 5HT and Dopamine	Causes Hypertension, Dyspepesai, Apoplexie	6, 8, 9, 11, 15
	Neostigmine, Guanethidine, Reserpine	Both are Antagonizers	Cancels therapeutic effect	11

Table 7.14 Interaction between Chinese Ready-made Medicines containing Chinese Herb Dan Shen (Salvia Miltiorrhiza) & Orthodox Drugs

Chinese Ready-made Medicines	Orthodox Drugs	Reasons	Results	Ref.
Break into a Smile	*	Laboratory experiments in rats indicate that Dan Shen treatment increases absorption rate and bioavailability but decreases clearance and prolongs elimination half life of warfarin. These changes are reflected in the exaggeration of pharmacological effects with consequential prolongation of prothrombin time. Patients who have been on chronic treatment with warfarin experience prolonged prothrombin time when Da Shen preparations are taken. But Dan Shen alone does not affect prothrombin time.		12, 18
Clear the Soul	*		Warfarin treatment decreases	20
Dan Shen Pian	丹参片			
Jade Spring	*			
Radio Support	*			
Red Stirring	*			
Stir Field of Elixir	*			
Wu Ji Bai Feng Wan	乌鸡白凤丸			
	Magnesium Oxide, Calcium Carbonate, Aluminium Hydroxide	These anti-ulcer drugs will form precipitated compound when combined with Dan Shen.	Hinder absorption.	7, 8 25 (P286)
	5 Fluorouracil, Cyclophosphamide, lomustine, Bleomycin	These are chemotherapy drugs. The use of Dan Shen at the same time will promote metastasis of tumor.	Destroys the therapeurtic effect of the drugs.	7, 8

* The samples do not have Chinese names

Table 7.15 Interaction between Chinese Ready-made Medicines containing Chinese Herb Dang Gui (Angelica Sinensis) & Orthodox Drugs

Chinese Ready-made Medicines	Orthodox Drugs	Reasons	Results	Ref.
Ba Zhen Wan 八珍丸	Warfarin		Laboratory experiments in rabbits indicate that Dang Gui treatment does not alter the pharmacokinetics of warfarin, but increases the prothrombin time at steady state of warfarin while plasma warfarin concentrations remain the same. This suggests that co-administration of Dang Gui at steady state of warfarin, the anti-coagulation effect of warfarin is exaggerated. Patients who have been on chronic treatment with warfarin experience prolonged prothrombin time when Dang Gui supplement is taken. But Dang Gui alone does not affect prothrombin time.	12, 20
Bend Bamboo				
Brighten the Eyes				
Brocade Sinews				
Bu Zhong Yi Qi Wan 补中益气丸				
Chemo Support				
Clear Lustre				
Da Bu Yuan Jian 大补元煎				
Dang Gui Si Ni Tang 当归四逆汤				
Du Huo Ji Sheng Tang 独活寄生汤				
Ge Xia Zhu Yu Tan 膈下逐瘀汤				
Glorious Sea *				
Gui Pi Wan 归脾丸				
Long Dan Xie Gan Tang 龙胆泻肝汤				
Ming Mu Di Huang Wan 明目地黄丸				
Qing Wei San 清胃散				
Radio Support *				
Red Stirring				
Ren Shen Yang Rong Wan 人参养荣丸				
Root the Spirit *				
Run Chang Wan 润肠丸				
Shi Quan Da Bu Wan 十全大补丸				
Si Wu Tang 四物汤				
Stir Field of Elixir *				
Strengthen the Root *				
Tang Feng Tong Sheng San 防风通圣散				
Wen Jing Tang 温经汤				
Wu Mei Wan 乌梅丸				
Wu Ji Bai Feng Wan 乌鸡白凤丸				
Xiao Yao Wan 逍遥丸				
Xue Fu Zhu Yu Tang 血府逐瘀汤				

* The samples do not have Chinese names

Table 7.16 Interaction between Chinese Ready-made Medicines containing Chinese Herb Yin Chen (Herba Artemisiae Capillaris) & Orthodox Drugs

Chinese Ready-made Medicines		Orthodox Drugs	Reasons	Results	Ref.
Yin Chen Tang	茵陈汤	Chloramphenicol	They are Antagonizers	Reduces the effect of the drugs	7, 8, 10
Yin Chen Wu Ling San	茵陈五苓散	Quinidine	Precipitation is formed	Reduces absorption	15

Section Three

Training, Research and Documentation

8. TRAINING OF PROFESSIONALS QUALIFIED IN BOTH ORTHODOX MEDICINE AND TRADITIONAL CHINESE MEDICINE

KELVIN CHAN

INTRODUCTION

Over the past decade, patients in the West have taken a great interest in seeking treatment of their illnesses from practitioners of alternative or complementary medicine. Complementary medicine includes a fairly wide range of various disciplines. Some of these are related to orthodox medical practice, such as chiropractic and osteopathy. Some are originated from traditional practices such as aromatherapy, homeopathy, medical (Western) herbalism, and traditional Chinese medicine (TCM, both acupuncture and Chinese herbal medicine) or traditional medical practice from other ethnic groups. Most of these belong to the second category. This category involves the administration of therapeutic remedies (with the exemption of acupuncture) for treatment of illnesses. TCM in the second category is an example where key issues on the contribution of this therapy to healthcare in the West can be identified. It has had a profound influence on health systems in the Chinese communities all over world. Such influence has also affected other non-Chinese communities in their demand of TCM as part of healthcare (Chan, 1996). One of the major reasons is that, as indicated in the Chapters 4 and 5, TCM has the advantage that written records of the use of herbal mixtures have accumulated over thousands of years. Chronic illnesses, such as atopic dermatitis, that are resistant to orthodox medical treatment respond to CHM medications. (Atherton *et al.*, 1992). This Chapter examines the current trends of popularity of complementary medicine among exisiting orthodox medical practice, in the West, with particular attention to traditional Chinese medicine. The emerging acceptance of using CHM products will add on the burden of orthodox medical (OM) practitioners' prescribing responsibility of OM drugs. In order to detect herb-drug interactions we need well-trained practitioners who are knowledgeable of both TCM and OM.

THE EMERGING ACCEPTANCE OF COMPLEMENTARY AND ALTERNATIVE MEDICINES IN ORTHODOX MEDICAL PRACTICE

In this era of advances in biomedical science and technology in the developed countries, it is surprising to note the public spends a large amount of their earnings on over-the-counter health products related to traditional complementary medicines such as herbal and homeopathic remedies. Complementary medicines or therapies in Europe and alternative medicines in North America probably refer to the similar areas of so called non-conventional therapies or unorthodox treatments. Most orthodox general practitioners (GPs) and their professional organisations in the past have not generally accepted the practice of these therapies. For example, in the UK the British Medical Association (1986) concluded in their report on 'Alternative Therapy', published in May 1986, many patients are "comforted and may be healed" when under the care of practitioners of alternative medicine. The report working party felt that for many therapies a formal trial would be quite inappropriate, as "many alternative approaches to medicine do not base their rational on theories which are consistent with natural laws as we understand them." They also commented that "While we have a duty of fairness to practitioners of alternative therapies, our long term duty to our patients is not to support what may be passing fashions, but to ensure for them the benefits of medicine in the future." Since the early 1990s the position in discussions both with the BMA and in the public has altered, and there is a rapidly growing interest in complementary medicine, both in the UK and other developed countries where orthodox medicine is the only accepted medical practice. This is evident in the subsequent updating BMA publication of the "Complementary Medicine: New Approaches to Good Practice" in 1993 and in the use of the term 'Complementary' instead of 'Alternative'. The Department of Health in UK has established a Secretariat to advise the profession and to develop policies on this issue. National survey of orthodox GPs indicated that many have now an 'open mind' to the value of some complementary treatments (GMSC, 1992). Patients are increasingly asking their orthodox GPs to identify those individuals who are competent and adequately trained to carry out complementary treatments for their illnesses.

Little is known about why patients in developed countries seek complementary therapies. More treatment time, gentle touch, and compassion that complementary therapies may employ are not the only reasons as these are also regarded as good bedside manners in orthodox medicine (OM). Untested assumptions may include the side effects of orthodox drugs, general dissatisfaction with orthodox treatment, chronic illnesses demanding more attention than patients receiving from orthodox general practitioners, and desperation of unsuccessful treatments etc. There is an urgent need to set up research programmes to test out these assumptions. Nevertheless, the growing concerns have been the quality, safety and efficacy of complementary treatments. These depend on both the qualification of the practitioners and the quality of the products used (Chan, 1996a). On the other hand the World Health Organisation (WHO) has pointed out 80% of the population in the developing countries depend entirely on their traditional medicines including mainly herbal products. This observation has drawn worldwide attention to look for ways and means of setting up rational approaches in order to establish procedures for controlling the quality, safety, and efficacy of traditional medical treatments.

It is obvious that in the coming 21st century, people will be more informed about medical products and knowledgeable about matters relating to their health in curing and preventing illnesses. They may demand good quality treatment from both orthodox as well as complementary medicine. The future professional should be knowledgeable on their patients' medications and be aware of possible treatment interactions as they may be given both treatments intentionally or unintentionally, and possibly taken both medications with or without informing the practitioner. The consequence of ignorance will lead to adverse reactions in most cases. Beneficial outcomes of intentional combined use will ascertain the advantages of proper integral treatment.

TRAINING OF PRACTITIONERS QUALIFIED IN BOTH OM AND TCM

The ultimate goal of restoring the patient's health using safe and effective treatments depends on the quality of both the practitioners and the treatments. With orthodox medicine (OM) these are controlled by legislation and regulatory requirements and recognised by professional bodies. Professional bodies of traditional Chinese medicine (TCM) practice would gain similar respect in the West if they were recognised like their counterparts in the East. The quality of TCM products should also be regulated; unless this is guaranteed, it will be very difficult to demonstrate their efficacy and safety. Thus only when the quality, efficacy and safety of these products are assured can one assess their role in health care. Acceptable systems of education and regulatory control in TCM comparable to those observed in the Far East are needed in order to achieve this goal. Although setting up these will take time, it is of paramount importance that these systems are needed to safeguard patients' well being. The practitioner, whether qualified in the East or West, who is in charge of looking after the patient's well being, should be aware of the situation of interactions in the unavoidable combination treatments. It will be interesting to note how professionals of TCM in the Far East communities and in the non-Chinese culture are trained to cope with the emerging problems.

TCM Education in the Far East

In Mainland China, national infrastructure for the control on education, training and practice of TCM practitioners is well set up (refer to Chapter 6). In 1956 when the nation decided to re-activate and promote education and practice of TCM, apart from OM universities and colleges, 4 initial city TCM universities (in Beijing, Chengdu, Guangzhou and Shanghai), later joined by Nanjing, were established. Presently, there are 27 university level TCM institutes consisting of 7 TCM universities (original 5 plus one in Heilungjiang and one in Shandong), and 20 provincial TCM colleges. Some vocational level colleges include 4 ethnic colleges and 184 vocation schools. These institutes are responsible for offering nationally controlled undergraduate degree courses in Medicine and Pharmacy of 5 to 7-year and 4-year duration respectively. TCM students have to study basic medical science subjects and clinical clerkship relevant to those taken by OM students. Upon graduation and subsequent internship they are qualified to prescribe both OM and TCM treatment. Students in the degree course for OM can take the option of at least one-year extra to study their chosen aspects of TCM (acupuncture or herbalism). Upon graduation and practical experience they are allowed to practise TCM treatment. The TCM Division (State Administration of TCM) of the Ministry of Public of Health (MPH) that also controls the practice of TCM monitors all courses of TCM. In each of the 27 provincial cities there is at least one research institute of TCM which is linked with local TCM hospitals for manufacturing, practice and research of various disciplines of TCM. Most hospitals are equipped with both orthodox and TCM pharmacies. Some hospitals have integrated departments with specialists in both TCM and orthodox medicine. Patients can choose either treatment. In orthodox hospitals, TCM outpatient departments are available for consultation.

Recently, nation-wide approach to concentrate the progress and development of TCM teaching and research has given 5 key tasks to the 6 key institutes. Thus Chinese Materia Medica was assigned to Chengdu University of TCM, Internal Medicine to Beijing University of TCM and Guangzhou University of TCM, Surgery to Shanghai University of TCM, Gynaecology to Hei Long Jiang University of TCM and Acupuncture to Nanjing University of TCM. Post-graduate courses from Masters to PhD level are available to encourage research and development in major universities and colleges. Students taking 5-year courses in OM can choose to take an extra year of TCM training. After graduation and internship training they are allowed to prescribe TCM treatment.

In Taiwan, at present all TCM practitioners qualify by either mainstream education (7-year course after secondary education or 5-year course after post-baccalaureate) offered at the China Medical College in Tai Chung. The structure of the degree course is similar to the ones in Mainland China including OM basic medical sciences subjects such as those attended by OM students (Anatomy, Biochemistry, Physiology, Pharmacology etc.). Since the late 1980s and early 1990s the older generation of TCM practitioners had to pass the special examination with 18 months practice training at the China Medical College in Taichung. This is the only TCM undergraduate institute in Taiwan with a separate TCM research institute. There are two other TCM-research institutes in Taipei involved in both research and postgraduate training. Similar integral practice of TCM and orthodox medicines occur in some hospitals. In addition there are also private TCM clinics serving the public on national health scheme.

In Hong Kong, part-time (mainly evening and week-end) courses of TCM are available in the private sector. These courses have not been recognised by the Government as professional qualification as TCM practice is not bound by any legal commitment of the government. Patients going to the TCM practitioners are on their own accord. Over the past few years both University of Hong Kong and Chinese University of Hong Kong offer post-graduate short courses (certificate type) due to the public demand for better quality of practitioners and CHM products. The Department of Health have made initiatives by organising Working Parties, consisting of various professionals, to look at the regulation of TCM products since 1991 and the rationalisation of the qualification of TCM practitioners since 1995. Recently, the Research Grant Council has given substantial amount of funding for research and development of TCM in Hong Kong even though biomedical science research and other physical sciences have always taken the lion share of the research funding. The latest development is centring on the introduction of courses at university level in collaboration with the Mainland universities.

In Japan, orthodox medical doctors who have received training in Kampo medicine (an oriental medicine with modified TCM approaches) can prescribe Kampo treatment and medications of TCM composite formulae. Toyama Medical & Pharmaceutical University offers the only undergraduate training of one year duration in the curriculum of the 6 year-OM medical degree course. Four research institutes in other parts of Japan provide postgraduate teaching and research of Kampo medicine. OM practitioners can get Kampo medicine qualification at these institutes. Research and development of Kampo medicine has been very advanced, in particular the areas of composite formulae used in ancient Chinese prescriptions. One of the top 4 pharmaceutical industries only manufactures Kampo prescription medications using GMP facilities as its only source of turnover.

Table 8.1 Early development of TCM in Europe and the UK

Date	Notable Events	Reference*
16th century	early knowledge of acupuncture was brought into Europe via connection with Dutch and English East India Co. Ist European text was compiled by Wiliem ten Rhyne	Rhyne, T., 1683
17th century	a comprehensive account of acupuncture & moxibustion was written that had great influence on German acupuncture development	Kaempfer, E. 1712
19th century	Colonisation of Far East countries allowed more acupuncture and related TCM herbal knowledge reaching the West.	

*Adopted from Goodman, J. (1992) Acupuncture research in Great Britain reported to date. A survey for Council for Acupuncture-UK. A paper presented to the conference of the world Federation of Acupuncture Societies, Rome, 1992; Report of the Board of Science & Education, the British Medical Association on *Alternative Therapy*, British Medical Association, 1986, Appendix II, *Acupuncture*, 93–105.

Training Courses of TCM in non-Chinese Communities

The most influential aspect of TCM in the Western Europe has been the realisation of the possible usefulness acupuncture in orthodox medical practice since the late 16th Century (Table 8.1). However the practice of acupuncture has never been accepted in the orthodox medical circle until the first half of the 19th century when it was applied by a number of medical practitioners. Medical acupuncturists seldom liased with non-medically qualified acupuncturists, despite the increasing number of the latter group. This expansion was witnessed by the setting up of institutes giving more intensive and structured courses than those organised exclusively for medical doctors. Thus, the British Acupuncture Association was founded in 1961 by a group of practitioners who studied acupuncture in need for adequate educational and ethical standards. Subsequently the British College of Acupuncture was set up in 1964 and other schools and professional societies were set up in the 1970s, 1980s and recently. (Table 8.2) At present there are five registers of acupuncture and related TCM herbalism and eight schools offering acupuncture and TCM herbalism in various parts of UK. Most of them offer 2 to 4 years part time courses with certificates or diplomas on graduation. Some of the trainees would travel to China or other Far east countries to attend post-graduate courses mainly in acupuncture and returned to UK as more qualified practitioners. However, in a recent directive from the Minister of Public Health in China said that 'Non-doctors who acquire some knowledge from a short term course should not practise TCM'. Students who are not medically trained will no longer be able to obtain the same certificate as those who are. This has been a way of tightening TCM courses to maintain comparable standard and quality of TCM practitioners (Tomlinson, 1996).

The Register of Chinese Herbal Medicine and the recently established Council for Acupuncture (from the previous Directory of British Acupuncturists in 1982) with five

Table 8.2   Some Private Professional Societies and Schools of Acupuncture and Related TCM in the UK*

Society/Register	Associated College/School	Approx. Year of Establishment
The Traditional Acupuncture Society, TAS	College of Traditional Acupuncture	1963
British Acupuncture Ass. & Register, BAAR	British College of Acupuncture	1964
International Register of Oriental Medicine, IROM	The International College of Oriental Medicine	1975/1972
British Acupuncture Council, (formerly Directory of British Acupuncturists), BAC	5 major acupuncture colleges/schools	1982/1995
Chung San Acupuncture Society, CSAS	Chung San Acupuncture School	1984
Eligible for BAC membership	Northern College of Acupuncture	1988
No Associated register	The London Academy of Oriental Medicine	1991
Association of Traditional Chinese Medicine	No affiliated colleges	1992
The Register of Chinese Herbal Medicine, RCHM	no affiliated colleges	Recent
The Register of Traditional Chinese Medicine, RTCM	no affiliated colleges	Recent
No Associated Register	The London School of Acupuncture & TCM	Recent
No Associated register	College of Integrated Chinese Medicine	Recent
No Associated register	The London College of Traditional Acupuncture	Recent

* Adopted from Jin, Y., Berry M.I., and Chan, K. (1995) Chinese Medicine in the UK. In: Proceedings of the Pharmacy Practice Research Practice Session, British Pharmaceutical Conference, University of Warwick, September, 1995, P26.

professional associations in 1994 indicated the profession's intention to work to maintain common standards of professionalism in the practice of TCM in the UK. Currently two university courses are being run in acupuncture in the UK. The supply of TCM herbs and products for the practice of the profession has been mainly dependent on import of these from the Far East. Regulations concerning import of these products at present are similar to those for control on food substances. However more comprehensive systems to control these may be introduced in the near future. Moreover, there is a shortage of TCM pharmacists in the West to safeguard the quality of imported CHM products.

The impact of alternative medicine in the USA took place very much later than in the European countries. Acupuncture and related TCM complementary medicines in the USA became popular only after the visit of Nixon to China in the early 1970s when China developed the open door policy. However the Chinese communities there have self-medicated or consumed CHM herbs as tonics regularly. A official survey (Eisenberg *et al.*, 1993) on the nation published by the New England Journal of Medicine in 1993 revealed that 30% of the population used unconventional therapies and 70% of the health budget was spent upon treating those individuals who also sought help from unconventional therapies for chronic illnesses such as cancer, hypertension and depression. In response to this observation the National Institutes of Health set up the Office of Alternative medicine in 1992. This Office's mission was to support research to investigate the effectiveness of alternative therapies and provide information about alternative practices. There are also institutes provide part-time tuition for acupuncture and related courses on part-time basis.

At present, it is obvious that the training of TCM practitioners is quite different between the East and the West. As far as relevance of herb-drug interactions is concerned, the main objective is to train competent TCM practitioners who are knowledgeable about OM drug use and OM practitioners who are aware of CHM products' contribution to therapy when confronting patients who are taking both therapies. This is to safe-guard the well being of the patients. Therefore practitioners with dual qualifications are needed in healthcare of the 21st century.

THE QUALITY ASSURANCE AND CONTROL ON CHM PRODUCTS

Increasing concern and fear has also been expressed to their unsupervised use, efficacy, toxicity and quality of these natural products as well as the legal responsibilities of practitioners. Inclusion of orthodox medications such as antibiotics, non-steroidal drugs and steroids in TCM patent products was not considered as a positive attribute of TCM in the West (Karunanithy & Sumita, 1991). The use of fake or wrong herbs has contributed a negative opinion about the safety and efficacy of TCM products (Vanhaelen *et al.*, 1994). Many popular and expensive TCM herbs are in short supply and inferior substitutes or fake crude herbs have been found in the UK market (Yu *et al.*, 1995, 1997). Thus the quality, efficacy, and safety of TCM natural products are jeopardised. This will certainly cast doubts on research in the search of new leads from single herbs and controlled clinical studies of composite prescriptions.

Products of natural origin present the pharmaceutical analyst with problems arising from the complex nature and the inherent variability of their constituents. As with orthodox pharmaceutical products, evidence of quality, efficacy and safety have to be presented for licensing purposes. Readers are referred to Tables 1.2 and 1.3 in Chapter One that compare the two kinds of pharmaceuticals and products. It can be seen that the quality of the natural products is complicated by the presence of complex and variable constituents whose therapeutic activity is often unknown. Pharmacopoeia and Regulations for controlling of medicinal plants and products used for TCM practice in China is available for standardisation, quality control and legal requirements (The Pharmacopoeia Commission of PR China, 1992, 1995; Provision For New Drug Approval, 1992) of both exports and imports of medicinal materials. It is likely that because of the popularity and demand of CHM materials there could be shortage of such materials and that irresponsible traders may be involved with the dealing of transaction there are poor quality and fake CHM herbs and products available in the herbal market. This will certainly affect the efficacy and safety of medications (Chan, 1995).

It is inevitable that interested parties including academic institutes, professional bodies and semi-government agents in the West are concerned with the quality of their imported CHM materials. Noticeably, academic and professionals have written separate monographs on CHM herbs in Germany since 1996 with the help of academics from China on the Editorial Board. (Four were available at the 2nd International Conference for Phytomedicines held in Munich, September 1996). The contents of these monographs are specifically tailored for the requirements for the control of medicinal plants in Germany with more identification assays and chromatographic patterns and are not appropriate for TCM use. In the United Kingdom, similar drive has been started to set up an Authentication Centre for International Use of Traditional Chinese Herbal Medicine by the Royal Botanic Gardens in Kew. The Director of the Royal Botanic Garden wrote, "With the rapidly growing popularity of TCM in the West, it has become increasingly important to verify the herbs used. This is because lack of regulation has meant that the identity and quality of herbs used can be highly variables. In some cases, this variability has given rise to safety concerns amongst the public, the western medical profession and sectors of the TCM industry itself. With it's long history of plant science and the resources of its vast herbarium, library, living collections and laboratories, the Royal Botanic Gardens, Kew is ideally suited to develop such a centre." (Royal Botanic Gardens, 1997).

DEVELOPMENT OF PROCEDURE FOR QUALITY ASSURANCE OF CHINESE HERBAL MEDICINAL PRODUCTS AVAILABLE FOR INTERNATIONAL USE

One cannot over-emphasise the importance of good quality assurance of any medications before safety and efficacy can be assessed in laboratory and clinical situations. It has been pointed out that the chemical constituents in TCM natural products are very complex and their curative effects are often due to the co-ordinating actions of several, quite often, unknown chemicals. Such complication makes scientific assessment of the quality, safety and efficacy of TCM products difficult (Chan, 1995). Evidently international interests on this issue cannot be dealt with just by simply putting import restriction on CHM or other herbs from other sources. Within countries among the European Union there is yet a need to work out a harmonisation on the regulations for import and export of herbal products. The dimension can be more difficult in the case of CHM herbs. Qualified CHM practitioners who know how to use CHM prescriptions and pharmaceutical professionals who are familiar with the background of processing CHM herbs are needed to formulate agreeable and simple QA procedures. Purely authentication, identification and pharmacognostical assessment, using all conventional analytical methods of single CHM herbs imported into any countries is not the answer. This is because of how CHM herbs are used in composite prescription formulae (refer to Chapters 4 and 5). Therefore in addition to all those standard operation procedures (SOP) for assaying herbal materials used according to Herbal Pharmacopoeia in any countries it is important that one should assess the bioactivities of the prepared CHM products.

It has been demonstrated successfully that chemical pattern recognition of analytical chromatographic peaks as physico-chemical discriminant indices should be linked with in vivo pharmacological activities as biological discriminant indices in a computing algorithm for assessing the quality of some popular CHM herbs (Chan, 1995, 1996b). It is believed that such an approach will give a more confident and scientific interpretation of the quality of source materials and finished products. In view of the difficulty of quality control of composite formulae, which have been proved clinically effective and included in the Chinese Pharmacopoeia, pattern recognition will be extremely useful for quality assessment and authentication purposes, in addition to those SOP required in the monographs.

To achieve development of procedures for the quality assurance of CHM products professionals who should possess experience or expertise of working on herbal products and orthodox drug would be better suited to make contribution. The training of these professionals may also include investigations on herb-drug interactions. Both clinicians and scientific professionals of these categories can work together in clinical and laboratory situations in order to safeguard patients' well being when OM and CHM treatments are involved.

REFERENCES

Atherton, D.J., Sheehan, M.P., Rustin, M.H., Whittle, B. and Guy, M.B. (1992) Treatment of atopic eczema with traditional Chinese medicinal plants. *Pediatric Dermatology*, **9**(4), 373–375.

British Medicial Association (1986) *Alternative Therapy*. BMA Board of Science and Education, British Medical Association, London, 1986.

British Medical Association (1993) *Complementary Medicine:New Approaches to Good Practice*. BMA Board of Science and Education, British Medical Association, London, 1993

Chan, K. (1995) Progress in traditional Chinese medicine. *Trends in Pharmacology*, **16**, 182–187.

Chan, K. (1996) *Critical assessment of traditional Chinese medicine*. A Fellowship Report submitted to the Winston Churchill Memorial Trust., London, April, 1996

Chan, K. (1996a) The role of complementary medicine in healthcare. *Biology*, **43**(2), 50–51.

Chan, K. (1996b) Quality assurance of natural products: Recent development and future directions in the UK and EU. A Plenary Lecture given at the Conference on "Quality Assurance and Evaluation of Traditional Chinese Medicinal Products", Hong Kong Baptist University, Hong Kong, 27–30 June, 1996.

Eisenberg, D.M., Kessler, R.C., Foster, C., Norlock, F.E., Calkins, D.R. and Debanco, T.L. (1993) Unconventional medicine in the United States. Prevalence, costs, and patterns of use. *New England Journal of Medicine*, 328(4), 246–252.

General Medical Services Committee (1992) *Your Choices For The Future: Results of the General Medical Services Committee survey* (Electoral Reform Society), London, 1992

Jin, Y. Berry M.I & K. Chan, (1995) Chinese herbal medicine in the UK. *Pharmaceutical Journal*, **255**(suppl), R37,

Karunanithy R. and Sumita, K.R. (1991) Undeclared drugs in traditional Chinese anti-rheumatoid medicines. *International Journal of Pharmacy Practice*, **1**, 117–119.

Provision for New Drugs Approval (1992) *Supplementary Stipulations and Revision of Issues Related to Traditional Chinese Medicine*. Beijing, China, Ministry of Public Health, 1992

Royal Botanical Gardens (1997) *Traditional Chinese Herbal Medicine: An authentication Centre for International Use*. A Funding Proposal, Royal Botanical Gardens, Kew, London, 1997.

The Pharmacopoeia Commission of PRC (1992) *Pharmacopoeia of the People's Republic of China*. GuangDong Science and Technology Press, GuangDong, China. English Edition, ISBN: 7-5359-0945-O/R 174.

The Pharmacopoeia Commission of PRC (1995) *Pharmacopoeia of the People's Republic of China*. GuangDong Science and Technology Press, GuangDong, China. Chinese Edition, 1995.

Tomlinson, R. (1996) China tightens up Traditional Chinese Medicine courses. *British Medical Journal*, **312**, 20

Yu, H. Zhong, S. Chan, K. and Berry, M.I. (1995) Pharmacognostical investigation on traditional Chinese medicinal herbs: Identification of four herbs from the UK market. *Journal of Pharmacy and Pharmacology*, **47**(12B), 1129.

Yu, H. Zhong, S., Berry, M.I and Chan, K. (1997) Pharmacognostical investigation on traditional Chinese medicinal herbs: Identification of six herbs from the UK market. *Journal of Pharmacy and Pharmacology*, **49**(suppl.), 212.

Vanhaelen, M., Vanhaelen-Fastre, R., But, P. and Vanberweghem, J.L. (1994) Identification of aristolochic acid in Chinese herbs. *Lancet*, **343**, 174.

9. RESEARCH AND DOCUMENTATION

KELVIN CHAN

INTRODUCTION

The incidence of drug-drug interactions has been the concern for clinicians treating patients on multiple drug regimens. Generally speaking the greater the number of drugs the patient takes the greater the likelihood that adverse reactions may result. It has been observed that in hospital and outpatient prescribing an interaction is reported when an average between 4 to 8 drugs are being taken by the patient (Glazener, 1992). The incidence is likely to be higher in the elderly patients because of the deteriorating hepatic and renal functions during the ageing processes that reduce elimination of drugs (Cadieux, 1989; Tinawi and Alguire, 1992). Knowing that two or three needed drugs can or will interact does not necessarily contra-indicate their use. Adverse reactions when occur due to combination therapy require adjusting doses rather then discontinuing needed therapy (Wright, 1992). Drug therapies of certain chronic diseases such as heart failure, coronary heart diseases and hypertension often involve more than one drug with different pharmacodynamic actions to achieve a satisfactory result without too many side effects. Sometimes, a drug used to treat an illness may cause side effects that have to be treated with an additional drug. For example the inclusion of ephedrine in some commercially available (over-the-counter) cough-mixtures or medications containing antihistamine is to counteract drowsiness caused by the latter drug. However prescribers' attention is needed to handle cases of drug-drug interaction involving OTC medications and prescribed drugs. Most of these interactions are predictable and avoidable from the known ingredients of the medications.

With the increasing popularity of complementary medicine that involves administration of usually unknown chemical entities such as CHM products, herbs of other sources, homeopathy, and aromatherapy, there will be a rise in the potential for adverse herb-drug reactions. Therefore studying these disciplines of biomedical science will become important aspects of the healthcare in the coming 21st century.

RESEARCH ASPECTS

Approaches on Research into Drug-Drug Interactions in Orthodox Medicine

Before looking into the complexity of interactions between herbal ingredients and orthodox drugs it is crucial to review steps that can be planned to investigate drug-drug interactions. The mechanisms involved in drug-drug interactions can be referred to Chapter 3. One should always bear in mind that only the clinically significant interactions are relevant to clinical practice. As a result of the focus on adverse drug interactions over the past 20 years, many of these are now predictable and unwanted reactions using drug combinations can be avoided by dosage adjustment of one or more of the interacting drugs. Unfortunately

Table 9.1 Some criteria considered as potential risks for occurrence of drug-drug interactions

- Drug-drug interactions of 2 or more drugs observed in clinical practice for confirmations
- Drugs with steep dose-response curve (a small change in concentration will lead to exaggerated effects)
- Drugs with small therapeutic range especially in combination dosage forms
- Drugs with problematic disposition or pharmacokinetics
- Drugs used for long term treatment having effects on drug cumulation, enzyme induction etc.
- Drugs prescribed simultaneously by several physicians intentionally or unintentionally
- Drugs self-medicated by patients
- Drugs showing genetic polymorphism in metabolic elimination (CYP2D6, CYP2C19 etc.)

many drug interactions that have been listed in the literature are neither meaningful nor helpful for clinical practice if they are not relevant. This is because many interactions are theoretically possible on the basis of in vitro investigations or animal experimentation that may not have been studied in patient situation. Some studies are based on healthy volunteer investigations or at non-therapeutic doses. The following headings describe possible steps one can initiate studies on drug-drug interactions

Criteria for Choosing Interaction Studies of Clinical Relevance

Before any studies are carried out, the project leaders should ascertain how valid the reported interaction is, and whether it is worthwhile to design a study to verify the importance of the reported or suspected interactions. Investigational studies of drug-drug interactions can be of predictive value if they mimic the clinical situation and they can be related to drug combinations and regimen that are practised in the clinic.

Drugs with problematic disposition and pharmacokinetics and those required for long-term treatment carry the higher risk of occurrence of possible clinically relevant interactions. Situations when patients self-medicate or on multiple drugs regimen also warrant investigations. The criteria summarised in Table 9.1 will be helpful to make a decision.

Types of Interaction Studies Relevant for Clinical Practice

Specific studies, based on the relevant criteria listed in Table 9.1, can be carried out during the development of new drugs (or CHM products, refer to later headings). These may be designed to measure certain biochemical or physiological processes or functions being affected by drug treatment with narrow therapeutic ratios. Table 9.2 gives examples of the pharmacological classes of drugs and respective processes involved for monitoring.

In general, clinical drug interaction studies should be performed during drug development with the standard drug treatment for the proposed indications and with drugs frequently co-administered with the new drug and for which clinically relevant interactions are known (Table 9.2).

Moreover, clinical interaction studies are indicated if the interactions: (a) are suspected from pre-clinical animal studies, (b) are expected from the physico-chemical properties (see Table 1.1 in Chapter One), (c) are expected from pharmacological properties, (d) are known from similar classes of compounds and (e) are observed during clinical trials.

Table 9.2 Pharmacological classes of drugs with clinical relevant interactions

Pharmacological Class	Functions to be monitored	Parametres
Antacids	formation of unabsorbable complexes	plasma levels of drug
Anti-arrhythmics	cardiac rhythm	ECG monitoring
Anti-asthmatics	respiratory stress	respiratory functions
Anti-coagulants	blood clotting or haemorrhagic crisis	prothrombin time
Anti-convulsants	uncontrolled epilepsy or oversedation	seizure frequency
Anti-diabetics	glucose homeostasis	blood glucose levels
Anti-hypertensives (β-blockers)	irregular blood pressure (BP)	monitoring BP
Cardiac glycosides	heart failure or over-digitalisation	monitor arrhythmia
Cytotoxic agents	over-suppression of immune functions etc.,	Check immune indices
H_2 receptor blockers	inhibition of drug metabolic elimination	Plasma levels
Psychotropic agents (particularly lithium, MAOIs)	hypertensive crisis	Check BP

The Timing of Clinical Interaction Studies for New Drugs

Generally, clinical interaction studies are performed during late phase 2 and phase 3 of clinical drug development after having obtained sufficient information on efficacy, safety and tolerability of the new drug. In exceptional cases interaction studies are carried out during the early stage of phase 2 clinical trial if co-administration of another drug is needed to minimise the patients' risk during the wide spread clinical investigation. This is especially crucial if the co-medication has a narrow therapeutic window or evidence obtained from initial screening (population pharmacokinetics and pharmcaodynamics) during phase 2/3 of the clinical trial. Results obtained under this circumstance of clinical interaction studies may be important for the decision to develop the new drug or not.

Actions to be Taken in Dealing with Interactions in Clinical Situation

In order to clarify an interaction as clinically significant it is necessary to test the interaction in a patient population and to simulate the clinical situation in which the drugs are given together as closely as possible. Unsuspected drug interactions should be observed and detected from the pharmacological and therapeutic information of the interacting drugs. Suspected drug interactions should be confirmed by appropriate clinical studies. Established drug interactions should be assessed for their incidence and clinical significance.

Unsuspected drug interactions: may be identified by intensive surveillance of patients receiving drug or combination of drugs. The surveillance programmes should include the following steps: (1) standard methods of prescribing, (2) recording of the administration of drugs, (3) operation of ward pharmacy systems whereby pharmacists scan all patients' prescriptions at ward level daily and subsequently ensure adequate supplies of drugs for the ensuing 24 hours. Pharmacists can readily identify patients receiving a specific drug or combination of drugs who can then be studied prospectively. If the interacting new drug or drugs in combination fall into the criteria as suggested in Tables 9.1 and 9.2, the clinical relevance should be investigated in a formal study as early as possible during clinical development. The mechanisms involved should be elucidated as soon as possible.

Suspected drug interactions: arise from clinical observations or pharmacological observations reported from literature. The suspected interaction can be investigated for hospital populations by applying epidemiological techniques to retrospective data based on good drug records. The object is to increase or decrease the suspicion and to indicate the most appropriate line for detailed prospective investigation to take.

Established drug interactions: require good documentation. For example, the ability of phenobarbitone to stimulate the metabolism of the oral anticoagulant, warfarin, and consequently decrease pharmacological effects of this drug has been well documented. To investigate the significance of this drug interaction a carefully planned study was carried out using carefully matched controls receiving warfarin but no phenobarbitone and patients receiving warfarin and phenobarbitone, the phenobarbitone group received on average significantly more warfarin. Therefore, the limitation of retrospective studies due to the inadequate medical records are reduced by prospective studies which required good records, the use of control groups and to be economical on selection on suspected or established drug interactions.

Design of Clinical Interaction Studies

It is not practical to evaluate all theoretically possible interactions for all drugs used clinically. A selection should be made for testing drugs for clinical interaction studies. In addition to consider groups of drugs that may be required for studies (see Table 9.1) certain criteria for selection should be considered. These may include severity of the diseases, choice of subjects (patients or healthy volunteers), drugs that undergo high first-pass metabolism, drugs showing interactions from in vitro metabolic studies or animal investigation, drugs predominately metabolised by one enzyme, target drugs showing genetic polymorphism in metabolic elimination (e.g.CYP2D6, CYP2C19) and drugs showing potential pharmacodynamic interaction profile from pharmacological mechanisms.

Study design with clear targets is necessary to determine whether the combined herb-drug effect is a true interaction or simply the result of additive therapeutic or pharmacological effects. An optimised protocol will help to obtain maximum information from experiments performed in a limited number of healthy volunteers or patients. Determination of plasma concentrations of the interacting drug(s) is needed to obtain pharmacokinetic and disposition parameters. Monitoring of clinical effects and changes of biochemical, haematological and physiological profiles of the patients under study will give the pharmacodynamic effects of the interacting drugs. These results may help explanation of possible pharmacokinetic and or pharmacokinetic-pharmacodynamic mechanisms of interactions. Table 9.3 summarises key points for the design of interaction studies.

Problems Involved in Investigative Drug Interactions in Clinical Practice

Over-reaction: In certain cases when the significance and importance of drug interactions is closely examined, the clinical problem presented by undesirable interactions between drugs has been vastly over-estimated and its applicability exaggerated. This may present two major difficulties to the general practitioners (GP). Firstly, the GP who prescribes the drugs to patients may become so confused after looking up all those tables for DI that

Table 9.3 Key points for consideration in designing interaction studies

- Clear targets and objectives with measurable observations and parameters
- Study protocol should include design of crossover, group comparison, randomisation etc.
- Study should be conducted using the most common administration route, e.g. oral route
- Monitoring both pharmacokinetics and pharmacodynamics parameters with probable correlation analyses
- Study should be conducted under steady state of medications. Parameters obtained will reflect true treatment picture as
  (1) the patient can act as his or her own control
  (2) any transient interactions can be detected (due to alteration of drug elimination process)
  (3) full time course of the interaction events can be traced
  (4) ascertain if the new drug is necessary for continuous treatment.

he himself may become the victim to the "Drug-interaction" anxiety syndrome. Secondly, a more probable outcome is a judgement by the GP that such lists do not agree with his clinical experience and that the whole concept of DI is only academic's exercise. It is only when an unexpected toxic effect or a decreased therapeutic effect is observed during actual clinical use of drugs, then the interaction is noticed. This may be too late.

Documentation and Reliability of Clinical Data: Many reports are based on single case or re-studies without further investigation into the frequency of occurrence of the severity of the interaction, the conditions under which the studies were carried out and the mechanism involved. This leads to misinformation. Uncontrolled observation is also misleading: For example, 10 years ago a single patient study led to the suggestion that chloral hydrate induced the metabolism of warfarin oral anticoagulant and therefore reduced the anticoagulant effect. In a prospective study of 500 patients, chloral hydrate increased the anticoagulant effect of warfarin in 54% of the patients. There was no evidence for the reduction of biological effect. In this controlled trial and laboratory study, the temporary potentiation was due to partial displacement of warfarin from albumin by trichloro-acetic acid, the major metabolite of chloral hydrate. But, some reviews or tabulations in the literature still report the interaction action of chloral hydrate with warfarin as clinically important.

Failure of communication: Communication gap exists between clinicians and other health professionals, one may not be aware of drugs prescribed for his patients by other doctors. Nowadays more organised system of information on drug use should be set up for a centralised co-ordination of dispatching information on the drug usage related problems and principles. This will help prescribers better informed and updated on drug related problems.

Disease state: Some interactions are likely to be modified by disease states but very little reliable information on this point is available. It is also difficult to differentiate between drug effects and manifestations of diseases. Nevertheless the effects of plasma protein displacement interactions are likely to be more marked in patients with hypo-albuminaemia. Cardiovascular diseases will invariably affect regional blood flow including the hepatic circulation thus affecting drug elimination by the liver. Renal dysfunction slows down elimination via the renal route thus lengthening elimination time and prolonging therapeutic or side effects of drugs.

Self-administration: Availability of drugs without prescriptions which patients acquire without informing the prescriber will influence current pharmacotherapy. Common examples are: ethanol, aspirin, cough mixture, nasal decongestants, antacid, etc.

Dietary habits: The influence of diet on drug actions has been observed leading to adverse effects during drug treatment (Cunningham and Smith, 1992). The mechanisms may involve antagonism or potentiation of endogenous substances or affecting the disposition (ADME) of the prescribed drugs leading to increased drug effects. For examples, cheese interacts with non-selective mono-amine oxidase inhibitors (MAOI) causes hypertensive crisis of drugs due to the increase in adrenergic activities caused by inhibition on the elimination of endogenous neurotransmitters. The presence of natural substances in grapefruit juice inhibits the metabolic elimination of some calcium antagonists that are prescribed for treatment of hypertension. One should note that the public considers some herbal products as food.

Individual variations: Genetically, there are individual differences in drug metabolism (Price Evans, 1996). Interaction may occur in some patients but not others. Drug interactions involving drug metabolism may vary greatly in different patients because of individual differences in the initial rate of metabolism and in the susceptibility to hepatic microsomal enzyme induction. For examples, phenylbutazone may potentiate warfarin effect in some patients but not in others. The inhibitory effect of isoniazid on phenytoin metabolism is only of clinical importance in low-acetylator of isoniazid.

Laboratory Approaches

Interactions from *in vitro* or *in vivo* animal studies should be extrapolated to clinical situations with caution and critical consideration. But such investigations are helpful for designing studies in man in terms of dosage regimen, etc. Nevertheless it is crucial to note that the absence of interactions in animal studies does not exclude the occurrence in man.

Predictability of drug interactions is sometimes possible. This is workable at least for known drugs or groups of drugs when a clinically relevant interaction has been detected and described and if the pharmacokinetic characteristics and mechanisms of drug actions are known. Carrying animal studies at this stage will be beneficial to understand and confirm clinical observations.

Thorough knowledge of the pharmacology, pharmacokinetics and biopharmaceutics of the interacting agents in healthy volunteer and animal studies would allow the predictability of drug interactions for new drugs or groups of drugs.

There may not be much choice for setting up or designing animal models that are appropriate to simulate clinical investigations. Although animal studies are of limited predicted value because of species variation; there may be an indication of qualitative value. There is a big gap between the extensive knowledge of drug interactions involving liver microsomal enzyme induction and inhibition in animals and the almost lack of information about similar mechanisms in man during the 1970s and early 1980s. Nowadays, biotechnological advances have enabled the isolation of different enzyme systems from the human liver that are useful for scientific investigations on interactions relating to liver metabolism of drugs (Gonzalez, 1997). Marker chemicals and some established endogenous metabolites are available for the purposes of studying enzyme inhibition and enzyme induction that form part of the mechanisms of drug-drug interactions involving dispositions and pharmacokinetics. Information on these aspects should be available during new drug development. It is not surprising that pharmaceutical industries will stop further development of a new drug if it is found to possess complicated metabolic elimination profiles. Nevertheless it is important to refine experimental systems and approaches for extrapolating data from the laboratory to the clinical situation. (Li and Jurima-Romet, 1997). Objective evaluation of laboratory and clinical data from observations of drug-drug interactions with clear understanding of the similarities and differences between these two sets of data can further advance technology, design and analysis. Sound scientific design with good communication among healthcare professionals and drug manufacturers together with good documentation will keep the incidence of adverse effects due to drug-drug interactions to a minimum. On the other hand, beneficial effects of combination treatments, balancing against side effects, such as those involved in chemotherapy, anti-microbial treatment, cardiovascular disease therapy etc., can be confirmed and properly catalogued.

APPROACHES ON RESEARCH INTO HERB-DRUG INTERACTIONS

Investigating the clinical efficacy of Chinese herbal medicinal (CHM) products in order to screen for new leads of pure chemical entities as potential drugs from plant extracts or other natural products using conventional extraction and approach has not produced much success. One of the many reasons for such a failure was that the research approach for orthodox screening and synthesis of compounds was not suitable for all medicinal plants which have demonstrated therapeutic activities when used traditionally (Chan, 1996). Nevertheless search for potential candidates as new leads for therapeutic agents from natural products has not been stopped (Zhu and Woerdenbag, 1995). On the other hand, clinical trials on the efficacy of traditional herbal remedies have supported the introduction of the following natural products. They are cranberry juice for urinary retention, garlic for reducing high blood pressure and cholesterol (Bordia, 1981), ginger for motion sickness and post-operative emesis (Grontved, 1988), tea-tree oil for acne, valerian for treatment of anxiety (Leathwood and Chauffard, 1985), feverfew for migraine prophylaxis (Waller and Ramsay, 1985) and a CHM herbal formula, for severe atopic eczema and related skin disorders that were resistant to orthodox treatments. The successful treatment of the skin disease, resistant to all possible orthodox therapies, by a combination prescription of 10 CHM herbs was carried out by a well designed double-blind clinical trial (Sheehan and Atherton, 1992). Each of these natural products contains several chemical entities, some of which are not yet identified. To carry out research on herb-drug interaction studies appears to be extremely challenging. It will be interesting to observe how the West appreciate medical research in assessing the efficacy and safety of herbal medicine before discussion on drafting protocols and designs for CHM herb-drug interaction.

Difficulty and Barriers towards Research in Herbal Medicine in the West

In the West, clinical and scientific research into the efficacy of herbal medicines in general using conventional methods has met difficulties (Mills, 1996). Three practical obstacles exist in pursuing good research for herbal medicines: (1) to obtain results with sufficient statistical weighting is expensive and laborious. Herbal medicine presently receives little or no funding from teaching hospitals, universities or industries in most organisations in the West. It is hopeful that through the Office of Alternative Medicines recently set up by the National Institute of Health in the USA some effort would be made to fill the gap of information on the quality, efficacy and safety of herbal medicine. In the UK the Medical Research Council has become more inclined towards funding well designed studies on complementary therapies. (2) Herbal medicinal products are complex mixtures with a vast amount of chemicals that may be pharmacologically active or inert. The composite formulae or prescriptions may have different properties from that of the single constituent acting alone. Acceptable models for investigation of herbal medicines from the orthodox medicine camp are not readily available. Herbal practitioners do not generally consider some orthodox models as relevant to assess herbal products that have been shown effective through time. (3) As mentioned in Chapters 4 and 5, the use of herbs and their effects on the body is not the same as usually understood for conventional medications. CHM medications are used to evoke healing responses in the body to rebalance body functions rather than to attack symptoms as orthodox medications do. Research of these types on CHM medications in the West is scarce. Clinical observations in the Chinese language are plentiful. This gap could be reduced in the near future with more international collaboration and understanding of methodology.

In his overview on research strategies of herbal medicines Mills (1996) gave some positive approaches that could be carried out on CHM medications in the West.

Observations of Clinical Studies Reported in Literature from the Chinese Language

Most of the interactions described in Chapter Seven are observations reported from clinical practice. They come from the integral approach of Chinese herbal medicine (CHM) and orthodox medicine (OM) to obtain the beneficial effects of combination treatment and some are adverse effects due to intentional or unintentional combination of CHM products and OM drugs. These observations are published in Chinese language. However information on potential interaction between OM drugs and homeopathics and herbal medicine is extremely scarce in the English language, although their use is gaining in popularity by consumers (Jurima-Romet, 1997). It has been indicated that information gap exists on herbal medicines and their potential for interaction with prescription and non-prescription medications. Evidently research in these areas are urgently needed in the West. However it is feasible to examine information of the clinical practice of TCM and OM in China and assess how herb-drug interactions can be studied using and adopting concepts from conventional pharmacological approaches, as presented above, with consideration of TCM principles of using CHM products.

Proposed Designs for CHM Medication-OM Drug Interaction Study

Therefore the most important step in dealing with CHM medications and OM drugs interactions is to obtain reliable sources of case studies. It may be necessary to accept initially the observed effects as suspected interactions and design studies to ascertain the finding by careful follow-up investigations within the patient group who needs the combination herb-drug treatment. All information on the interacting OM drugs stated in Tables 9.1 to 9.3 should be taken into account and considered as drug-herb interaction design. Consideration should include the TCM information on the CHM medications and their reported conventional pharmacological group functions (see Appendices 1 to 3 for classifications of CHM single herbs and prescriptions). Using this approach it is possible to adopt study design from the drug-drug interaction protocol only for those needed for patients. It is considered unethical to test on healthy volunteers for such study. Laboratory investigations will be needed to ascertain clinical observations.

Design for Interaction Study of Beneficial Effects

Using Case 1 of Category 5 'Reducing adverse effects due to OM chemotherapy during treatment of cancers with CHM medications' given in Chapter 7 as an example one can design a reasonable study. In the study reported by Rao *et al.* (Chapter 7 Part one, Category 5 case 1), the indications given for significant successful reduction of side effects were the general well being of the patients with stomach cancer on combination of chemotherapy and Sheng Xue Tang, SXT (literally means decoction or recipe producing new blood components). The results as reported could be more significant and convincing if other measure outcomes were explored and included in the trial. This might be due to the limited design and certain facilities that were not available during that study. It was obvious that the chemotherapy with MFV (methotrexate, fluorouracil and vinblastine) should not be stopped throughout treatment as decided by the oncologist, the co-administration of SXT would help to alleviate syndromes, due to adverse effects of the MFV treatment, as diagnosed by the TCM methodology.

   If this trial were to be repeated according the present suggested design here, it will include several entry requirements and other outcome measures with better statistical assessment. The 81 late stage gastric cancer patients could be divided into 3 groups of 21 each for 3 different treatments of MFV chemotherapy, MFV chemotherapy plus SXT decoction and MFV chemotherapy plus placebo decoction respectively. Details of design consideration are summarised below:

Trial Conditions and Procedure:

(1) Inclusion of a placebo preparation or decoction should give a better outcome of a controlled trial. A decoction similar in colour, smell but without the TCM effects could be prepared. The successful controlled trial in the atopic eczema study (Sheenan and Atherton, 1992) also included a placebo to increase the trial's confidence level of significance.

(2) Entry by randomisation of number of patients into the three treatment groups was a better design. Thus the 'Chemotherapy plus Sheng Xue Tang' group and the 'Chemotherapy plus Placebo Tang' could be compared with the Chemotherapy group only.

(3) Pre-chemotherapy profiles of clinical biochemistry and haematology and kidney and liver function of all patients should be available and recorded accordingly together

with other parameters for assessment of well being. The well being measurements should be administered by trained persons based on properly designed questionnaires. The person making the assessment should be blinded of both treatment groups.

(4) Measurement of adverse effects should also be performed with thoroughly designed protocol and recorded without biased remarks or comments. Same procedures should be administered for every patient.

(5) Run-in steady state of basic chemotherapy treatment should be achieved by measuring the pharmacokinetic parameters of the chemotherapy drugs during the first week before giving the SXT or Placebo Tang. Evaluation of pharmacokinetics of the chemotherapy drugs should commence simultaneously.

(6) Determination of pharmacodynamics and pharmacokinetics after steady state has attained should be carried out. Observation of adverse side effects and improvement or deterioration of blood picture and other related. Indices ahould be recorded.

Assessment of Outcomes: The possible outcomes may be as follows:

(1) If the SXT decoction is effective to reduce adverse effects of the MFV chemotherapy such as prevention of hair loss due to OM drugs, improving overall well being due to the immuno-protective or -stimulant actions of the CHM preparation, the confidence level of the significance will be higher due to the randomisation and inclusion of a placebo. The clinical biochemistry and haematology reports and kidney and liver function tests would be favourable. These data are essential indications how the body reacts to the combination treatment.

(2) The pharmacokinetics of the 3 cytotoxic drugs could be altered due to the complexity of the unknown chemicals in the SXT and placebo preparations. This alternation could only be detected if the disposition of these OM drugs were followed during the trial.

Figure 9.1 illustrates a summary of these points to be included in the trial.

Design for interaction studies of adverse effects

Similar precautions and consideration should be observed as for studying drug-drug interactions when investigating herb-drug interactions. Because of the fact that many known and unknown chemical entities are involved in herbal products it is not unreasonable to consider them as special food substances with the understanding that they are more potent and possibly toxic than daily consumed food substances. Adverse effects may be observed if OM drugs belonging to those listed in Tables 9.1 and 9.2 are co-administered with interacting CHM herbal products. The scheme (Figure 1) suggested for studying beneficial effects of herb-drug interaction could be applied to study herb-drug interactions in general. The following headings are considered for discussion.

Difficult situation involving ethical issues

There are certain ethical considerations and limitations in carrying out investigation on herb-drug interactions leading to adverse reactions in clinical situation. Each clinical interaction study requires a strict benefit-risk estimation, which takes into consideration

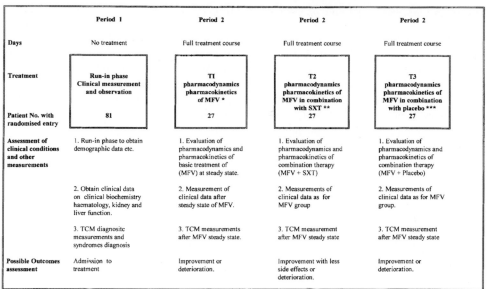

	Period 1	Period 2	Period 2	Period 2
Days	No treatment	Full treatment course	Full treatment course	Full treatment course
Treatment	**Run-in phase Clinical measurement and observation**	**TI pharmacodynamics pharmacokinetics of MFV ***	**T2 pharmacodynamics pharmacokinetics of MFV in combination with SXT ****	**T3 pharmacodynamics pharmacokinetics of MFV in combination with placebo *****
Patient No. with randomised entry	81	27	27	27
Assessment of clinical conditions and other measurements	1. Run-in phase to obtain demographic data etc.	1. Evaluation of pharmacodynamics and pharmacokinetics of basic treatment of (MFV) at steady state.	1. Evaluation of pharmacodynamics and pharmacokinetics of combination therapy (MFV + SXT)	1. Evaluation of pharmacodynamics and pharmacokinetics of combination therapy (MFV + Placebo)
	2. Obtain clinical data on clinical biochemistry haematology, kidney and liver function.	2. Measurement of clinical data after steady state of MFV.	2. Measurements of clinical data as for MFV group	2. Measurements of clinical data as for MFV group.
	3. TCM diagnositc measurements and syndromes diagnosis	3. TCM measurements after MFV steady state.	3. TCM measurement after MFV steady state	3. TCM measurement after MFV steady state
Possible Outcomes assessment	Admission to treatment	Improvement or deterioration.	Improvement with less side effects or deterioration.	Improvement or deterioration.

*   MFV = Methotrexate, Fluouracil, Vinblastin
**   SXT= Sheng Xue Tang (a CHM decoction of 8 herbs)
*** Placebo = a decoction of similar colour and taste but no SXT activity

Figure 9.1   Study for drug interaction studies in cancer patients.

of all laboratory and previous clinical observations. For example, Dang Gui (*Angelica Sinesis*), a CHM herb, is a popular herb for inclusion in home-made soup as a tonic. It was reported that patients, who were on steady state oral anti-coagulant (warfarin) treatment in the hospital after surgical operation of deep vein thrombosis, experienced bleeding crisis after taking Dang Gui-chicken tonic soup during convalescence at home. The adverse effect was confirmed in a laboratory observation (Lo *et al.*, 1995), in which the investigation was carried out in rabbits with single dose and under steady state conditions. Two of the rabbits died from excess bleeding three days after oral administration of the Dang Gui aqueous decoction at warfarin steady state. Dang Gui itself does not affect the prothrombin time and the pharmacokinetics of single dose or steady state of warfarin.

One way to substantiate the clinical observation would be to monitor all warfarin taking patients' steady state plasma warfarin and their prothrombin time when they self-medicate Dang Gui tonic soup for all reported cases after their re-admission to the hospital for observation. Good case history taking will be most essential. Patients under care would most probably be given an altered dosage regimen after stopping Dang Gui intake and the warfarin steady state level would be re-established at optimal with controllable prothrombin time.

The Ethical Committee may not approve studies in volunteers to confirm the pharmacodynamics effects and pharmacokinetics of warfarin during co-administration of Dang Gui.

Systematic laboratory studies of herb-drug interactions

Difficulty in studying clinical interactions in patients or healthy volunteers together with a general lack of information in the English language on the risk of CHM product-orthodox drug interactions necessitates to consider various types of laboratory approaches to screen combination CHM and OM medications. Some studies have reported the combined effects of CHM products with OM drugs reducing the dose and side effects of OM drugs (see accounts on beneficial effects in Chapter 7; Tani, 1989; Mizuno *et al.*, 1988). Only very few systematic laboratory studies have been reported on the effects of CHM products on the kinetics and dynamics of OM drugs (Lin, 1991).

It is feasible to set up laboratory protocol to screen commonly prescribed CHM products against those groups of OM drugs with potential adverse effects when combined with other substances (see Tables 9.1 and 9.2). Many *in vivo* animal models can be used to screen drug interactions between herbs and drugs. Pharmacokinetic and pharmacodynamic correlation may be achieved using these *in vivo* models. Pharmacokinetic clearance of OM drugs in presence of CHM products can be studied using *in vivo* model. The data obtained are useful qualitative guidelines for clinical studies.

In vivo models for interaction studies of CHM products and OM drugs involving drug metabolism enzymes (DME)

All CHM products should be studied using *in vivo* models to obtain data on pharmacokinetics and pharmacodynamics of interacting OM drugs. This is because of the presence of many known and unknown chemicals in the CHM preparations. *In vitro* or *in situ* models for studying metabolic clearance using human liver slices or hepatocytes will not be appropriate. The biotransformation of OM drugs is an important determinant of efficacy, duration of action and toxicity and can be assessed in presence of the CHM co-administration. The DME system, cytochrome P_{450}, can be induced or inhibit by the presence of CHM chemicals. Therefore the therapeutic or adverse effects of the OM drug can be affected. The activities of the DME system can be monitored by in term of concentrations of certain endogenous chemical such as 6-beta hydroxycortisol (6OHC) in the urine. This urinary excretion is an index of hepatic cortisol oxidation, and has been used as a non-invasive clinical test for enzyme induction (if the urinary excretion is greater then control) and inhibition (if the urinary excretion is less than control). This is particularly appropriate for monitoring the cytochrome P450IIIA3 family of DME as most drugs are eliminated via this enzyme. The endogenous steroid in urine is determined using monoclonal antibody-based ELISA method. The 6OHC- specific monoclonal antibody based ELISA assay can be utilised in patients who are taking the combination treatment in order to ascertain if the metabolic elimination of OM drugs is affected by CHM products.

DOCUMENTATION ASPECTS

OM practitioners and the public have expressed the concern and fear of CHM products causing toxicity. Yet reported cases of toxicity often give no information on the prescribed crude herbs or CHM products, pre-treatment profiles of patients' biochemistry, haematology, liver and kidney functions and OM medications. This can only lead to difficulty in drawing clear conclusions. Some other reported cases of toxic reactions due to CHM products have involved unqualified practitioners including OM practitioners who have no proper training in TCM. These can be related to poor documentation of reporting incidents of adverse reactions. Some of these reported adverse reactions could be consequences of CHM product-OM drug interactions.

A Centralised Co-ordination for Records of Adverse Drug Reactions (ADRs)

In handling adverse reactions of OM drugs well-established reporting schemes have been in operation in some developed countries. The author is familiar with schemes operating in the UK and Australia. The intention is to describe briefly these two schemes and make suggestions and modifications for use in recording and reporting adverse reactions involving herb-drug interactions. A centralised co-ordinating effort will be needed for quality information to make decision on all medications regarding restriction in use, reduction in dose, or special warnings and precautions.

The Yellow Card Scheme: The Committee on Safety of Medicines working with the Medicine Control Agency has established the Yellow Card Scheme (Rawlins, 1988, 1988a) for reporting adverse reactions of medications since 1964. It receives reports of suspected ADRs directly from doctors, dentists, coroners, and pharmacists and indirectly through pharmaceutical companies. It is the UK Adverse Drug Reactions Reporting Scheme. These received reports are placed on a specialised computer system, Adverse Drug reactions On-line Information Tracking (ADROIT) to facilitate rapid processing and analysis. The scheme has been critically important in monitoring drug safety in normal clinical practice, increasing knowledge about known adverse reactions, and acting as an early warning system for the identification of previously unrecognised adverse reactions. Figure 9.2 illustrates the organisation and operation of the Scheme including collection of reports of suspected adverse reactions, data processing, verification and confirmation of information, and dispatching of advice etc. The data received from reports of suspected ADRs will be analysed and presented and dispatched via the 'Current Problems in Pharmacovigilence' which is distributed to all doctors, dentists, coroners and pharmacists 3 to 4 times a year.

Obviously the accuracy of initial source of information of the suspected adverse reactions is extremely important. Guidelines on reporting are given. Table 9.4 shows a general format of reporting suspected adverse reactions arisen due to CHM medication-OM drug interaction proposed for action by the author. It is also a suggestion for TCM and OM practitioners' Good Clinical Practice to self-regulate until a similar scheme is accepted by appropriate health organisations in any countries that such a scheme is considered for monitoring. It is adopted from the UK Yellow Card Scheme reporting card issued by the Scheme operators. It is understood that the present UK Scheme also welcomes inclusion of suspected adverse reactions due to herbal medications. Table 9.5 listed categories of 'Adverse Reactions' considered serious for reporting as specified in the UK Yellow Card Scheme. In general, serious reactions include those that are fatal, life-threatening, disabling, incapacitating or that result in or prolong hospitalisation.

The Blue Card System: The Adverse Drug Reactions Advisory Committee (ADRAC), a subcommittee of the Australian Drug Evaluation Committee, encourages the reporting

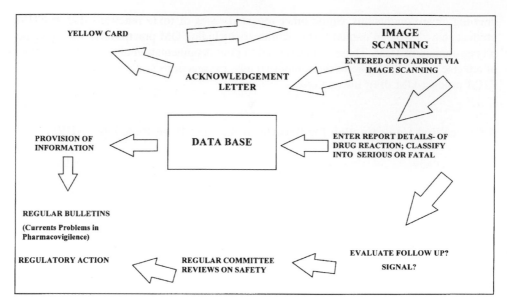

Figure 9.2   Handling of reported data in the yellow card scheme by ADROIT (Adverse Drug Reactions On-Line Information Tracking). Approval for reproduction is obtained from CSM, UK.

of all Suspected Adverse Reactions to drugs or other medical substances, including herbal, traditional or alternative remedies. Table 9.6 gives a summary of items considered relevant for reporting to the ADRAC. Regular Australian Adverse drug Reactions Bulletin is distributed to appropriate healthcare professionals for their information free of charge. A modified 'Blue Card' is proposed to deal with reporting or recording interactions between CHM products and OM drugs for TCM and OM practitioners' self-regulatory practice (Table 9.7).

Other developed countries may also have similar establishments who would deal with ADRs reporting. Whatever systems are available, it is possible to modify them for reporting and recording ADRs due to interactions between CHM medications and OM drugs.

Establishing A Data Base for CHM Medication-OM Drug Interactions

It is hoped that for Good Clinical Practice practitioners of TCM or OM who prescribe CHM medications would make use of adopting a system of recording and reporting the incidence of ADRs and beneficial effects of interactions between CHM medications and OM drugs. It is probable to start a self-regulating system within their own academic/professional organisation and up grading to a nationally recognised body for TCM practice. Because of the differences in diagnosis and treatment approaches between TCM and OM, the integration concept in treatment cannot be put into practice unless there are qualified practitioners of both disciplines. The information obtained from the reporting system on interaction ADRs may not be analysed properly and accordingly. Such report analysis

Table 9.4 *A suggestion for reporting suspected adverse reactions due to interactions of Chinese Herbal Medication Products and Orthodox Medicine Drugs.

All information are kept as confidential records
Do not put off reporting because some details are not known

REPORTER: HEALTH CARE PROFESSIONALS

Name _____

Professional _____

Address _____
_____
_____

Telephone _____

Speciality _____

Signature: _____ Date: _____

OM PRACTITIONERS/TCM PRACTITIONERS

Name _____

Professional _____

Address _____
_____
_____

Telephone _____

Speciality _____

Has this case been discussed with
the consultant / GP   Yes ☐   No ☐

PATIENT'S DETAILS   Sex **M** ☐   **F** ☐   Weight Kg [_____]

SURNAME _____   Hospital if relevant _____

Other names _____   Hospital Number _____   Date of birth (or age) _____

SUSPECTED CHINESE HERBAL MEDICINAL PRODUCTS

Give brand name of formulae or herbs	Route	Daily dose	Date started	Date stopped	Therapeutic indication
_____	_____	_____	__/__/__	__/__/__	_____
_____	_____	_____	__/__/__	__/__/__	_____

ORTHODOX DRUGS TAKEN IN THE LAST 3 MONTHS INCLUDING SELF-MEDICATION

Give brand if known. Write None if no other drugs has been taken	Route	Daily dose	Date started	Date stopped	Therapeutic indication
_____	_____	_____	__/__/__	__/__/__	_____
_____	_____	_____	__/__/__	__/__/__	_____
_____	_____	_____	__/__/__	__/__/__	_____
_____	_____	_____	__/__/__	__/__/__	_____

SUSPECTED REACTIONS

Is the patient hospitalised   Yes ☐
because of the reaction?   No ☐

			Date reaction started	Date reaction ended	Outcome eg. fatal recovered, continuing
_____	_____	_____	__/__/__	__/__/__	_____
_____	_____	_____	__/__/__	__/__/__	_____
_____	_____	_____	__/__/__	__/__/__	_____
_____	_____	_____	__/__/__	__/__/__	_____

Relevant additional information including medical history, investigations, known allergies, suspected drug interactions. For congenital abnormalities state all other drugs taken during pregnancy and the LMP. Please attach additional pages if necessary _____
_____   ● If you would like information about other reports associated
_____   with the suspected drug , tick here☐

---

*   Adopted from the Yellow Card Scheme for Reporting ADRs, UK (Approval for adoption is obtained)

Table 9.5   Some examples of serious adverse reactions (adoption from UK Yellow Card Scheme is approved).

Blood	**Gastrointestinal**	**Renal**
Bone marrow dyscrasias	Colitis	Renal dysfunction
Coagulopathies	Haemorrhage	Urinary retention
Haemolytic anaemias	Hepatic cirrhosis	
	Hepatic dysfunction	**Reproduction**
Cardiovascular	Hepatic fibrosis	Abortion
Arrhythmias	Ileus	Antepartum haemorrhage
Cardiac arrest	Pancreatitis	Congenital abnormalities
Cardiac failure	Perforation	Eclampsia, pre-eclampsia
Cardiomyopathy	Peritonitis (inc. fibrosing)	Infertility
Circulatory failure	Pseudo-obstruction	Uterine haemorrhage, perforation
Hypertension		
Hypotension	**Immunological**	**Respiratory**
Myocardial	Anaphylaxis	Alveolitis (allergic, fibrosing)
ischaemia/infraction	Arteritis	Bronchospasm (inc. exacerbation)
Sudden death	Drug fever	Pneumonitis
	Graft rejection	Respiratory failure
Central nervous system	Lupus syndrome	Thromboembolism
Anorexia nervosa	Polyarteritis nodosa	
Catatonia	Vasculitis	**Skin**
Cerebrovascualr accident		Angiodema
Coma	**Malignancy**	Bullous eruptions
Confusional state	Any	Epidermal necrolysis
Dependence		Exfoliation (generalised)
Depression	**Metabolic**	
Epilepsy	Acidosis	**Special senses**
(inc. exacerbations)	Adrenal dysfunction	Cataract
Extrapyramidal reactions	Hyperalcaemia	Corneal opacification
Hallucinations	Hyperkalaemia	Glaucoma
Hyperpyrexia	Hypokalaemia	Hearing loss
Intracranial hypertension	Hyponatraemia	Vestibular dysfunction
Myasthenia	Pituitary dysfunction	Visual loss
Myopthies	Porphyria	
Neuropleptic malignant syndrome	Thyroid dysfunction	
Neuropathy		
Psychosis	**Musculoskeletal**	
Withdrawal syndrome	Arthropathy	
	Aseptic bone necrosis	
	Osteomalacia	
	Pathological fracture	

should examine the reasons for administering CHM medications. It is because of these reasons that a separate ADR monitoring system for data concerning CHM-OM interactions would be more appropriate and useful. Tables 9.4 and 9.7 are suggested as possible forms for setting up this separate system of reporting. The popularity of using CHM medications in the future, when the quality of both TCM-OM (or OM-TCM) practitioners and CHM medications are guaranteed, would contribute towards different aspects of providing good healthcare for patients.

Table 9.6 Items for inclusion in the reporting of Adverse Drug Reactions (Blue Card) to the Adverse Drug Reaction Advisory Committee (ADRAC), Australia; approval for reproduction is obtained.

- All suspected reaction to **NEW DRUGS** especially **DRUGS OF CURRENT INTEREST**.
- All suspected drug interactions.
- Reactions to other drugs that are suspected of significantly affecting a patient's management, including reactions suspected of causing.
  - Death
  - Danger to life
  - Admission to hospital
  - Prolongation of hospitalisation
  - Absence from productive activity
  - Increased investigational or treatment costs
  - Birth defects

Reports of suspected adverse drug reactions are best made by using a prepaid reporting form ("Blue Card") which is available from the Adverse Drug Reactions Section.

Table 9.7 *A suggestion of reporting suspected adverse drug reaction involving interactions of Chinese Medicinal Products and Orthodox Medine Drugs

(Note: Identification of Reporter, Patient and Institution will remain **Confidential**)
Patient (Initials ot Record No. Only)

Age: Height:
Sex: Weight:

Adverse Reaction Description: Date of Onset of Reaction: /   /

All Chinese Herbal Medicinal products and Orthodox Medicine Drugs Prior to Reaction Asterisk Suspected Medication(s) (Please use trade names)	Daily Dosage and Route	Date Begun	Date	Reason for use Stopped

Treatment (of reaction):
Outcome: Recovered ☐   Date of Recovery: /   /
   Not Yet Recovered ☐   Unknown ☐   Fatal ☐   date of Death   /   /
Sequelae: No ☐   Yes ☐ (describe)
Comments (eg. relevant history, allergies, previous exposure to this drug):
Reporting Doctor ☐   or Pharmacist ☐   Others ☐ (Please tick)
Name:
Address:
                                    Signature_____ /   /
Return Form(s) To University Department on Professional Assocaiation of Traditional Chinese Medicine
Address: Fax:
*Adopted from the Blue card System of the ADRAC, Australia (Approval is obtained).

REFERENCES

Bordia, A. (1981) Effects of garlic on blood lipids in patients with coronary heart disease. *American Journal of Clinical Nutrition*, **34**, 2100–2103.

Cadieux, R.J. (1989) Drug interactions in the elderly. *Post-Graduate Medicine*, **86**, 179–186.

Chan, K. (1996) The importance of natural products in drug development. In: *Proceedings of the 7th South East Asian & Western Pacific Regional Meeting of Pharmacologists*, The Philippine Society of Experimental & Clinical Pharmacology, Manila, November, 1995, 480–483.

Cunningham R.K. and Smith C.M. (1992) Interactions: Drug allergy; Drug-drug; Drug-food In: Textbook of Pharmacology, Smith C. and Reynard, A.M. (editors), Suanders, International Edition, 1992, pp 1090-1103.

Glazener, F.S. (1992) Adverse drug reactions. In: Melman, K.L., Morreli, H.F., Hoffman, B.B., Nierenberg, D.W.(eds), Melman and Morreli's *Clinical Pharmacology: Basic Principles in Therapeutics*. McGraw-Hill, Inc., pp. 977–1011.

Grontved, A. *et al.* (1988). Ginger root against seasickness: a controlled trial on the open sea. *Acta Otolaryngology*, **105**, 45-49.

Gonzalez, F.J. (1997) Overview of experimental approaches for study of drug metabolism and drug-drug interactions. In: *Advances in Pharmacology,* Vol. 43, Academic Press, 1997, 255–278.

Jurima-Romet, M. (1997) Drug Interactions: Perspectives of the Canadian Drugs Directorate. In: Advances in Pharmacology, **Vol. 43**, Academic Press, pp. 239–254.

Leathwood, P.D. and Chauffard, F. (1985) Aqueous extract of valerian reduces latency to fall asleep in man. *Planta Medica*, **54**, 144–148.

Li, P.L. and Jurima-Romert, M. (1997) Overview: Pharmacokinetic Drug-drug interactions. In: *Drug-drug interactions: Scientific and regulatory perspectives*, Academic Press, International Edition, pp. 1–6.

Lin, S.-L., Hou, S.-J., Wu, W.-H., Chen, S-M, and Young, T.-K. (1991) Effect of traditional Chinese Herbal Medicines on the pharmacokinetcs of Western Drugs in SD rats of different ages: 1. Aminophylline-Tin Chuan Tang and aminophylline-Hsiao Ching Long Tang. *Journal of Pharmacobiological Dynamics*, **14**, 201–206.

Lo, A.C.T., Chan, K., Yeung, J.H.K. and Woo, K.S. (1995) Dang gui (Angelica sinesis) affects the pharmacodynamics but not the pharmacokinetics of warfarin in rabbits. *European Journal of Drug Metabolism and Pharmacokinetics*, **20**, 41–46.

Mills, S. (1996) Herbal medicines: research strategies. In: *Fundamentals of Complementary and Alternative Medicine*, Churchill Livingston, International Edition, pp. 394–407.

Mizuno, M., Iinuma, M., Yasuda, K. and Kawada, I. (1988) Combined effect of Chinese medicine and western drug. *Ann Proc. Gifu Pharm. Univ.*, **37**, 18–28.

Price Evans, D.A. (1993) *Genetic factors in drug therapy: Clinical and molecular pharmacogentics*, Cambridge University Press, UK, 1993.

Rawlins, M.D. (1988) Spontaneous reporting of adverse drug reactions I: The data. *British Journal of Clinical Pharmacology*, **26**, 1–5.

Rawlins, M.D. (1988a) Spontaneous reporting of adverse drug reactions II: Uses. *British Journal of Clinical Pharmacology*, **26**, 7–11.

Sheehan, M.P. and Atherton, D.J.A. (1992) A controlled trial of traditional Chinese medicinal plants in widespread non-exudative atopic eczema. *British Journal of Dermatology*, **126**, 179–184.

Tani, T. (1989) The Chinese herbal medicines to prevent the side effects of western drugs. *Medicine Drug Journal (Japan)*, **25**, 1987–1987.

Tinawi, M. and Alguire, P. (1992) The Prevalence of drug interactions in hospitalised patients. *Clinical Research*, **40**, 773A.

Waller, P.C. and Ramsay, L.E.(1985). Efficacy of feverfew as prophylactic treatment of migraine. *British Medical Journal*, **291**, 1128

Wright, J. M. (1992) Drug interactions. In: Melman, K.L., Morreli, H.F., Hoffman, B.B., Nierenberg, D.W.(eds), Melman and Morreli's *Clinical Pharmacology: Basic principles in therapeutics*. MaGraw-Hill, Inc., pp. 1012–1021.

Zhu, Y.-P., and Woerdenbag, H.J. (1995) Drug development from traditional Chinese medicine. *Pharmacy World & Science*, **17**, 103–112.

APPENDICES

LILY CHEUNG

This Section contains 3 Appendices

Appendix One gives lists of commonly used Chinese medicinal herbs that are classified according to traditional Chinese medicine actions. There are 18 separate categories.

1. Diaphoretics (Herbs for treating exterior syndrome,
2. Heat-clearing herbs,
3. Purgative Herbs
4. Aromatic herbs for removing dampness
5. Herbs for inducing diuresis and excreting dampness
6. Antirheumatic herbs (expelling wind and dampness)
7. Herbs for warming interior
8. Herbs for inducing resuscitation
9. Sedative and tranquilizer herbs
10. Herbs for calming the liver to check endogenous wind
11. Herbs with antitussive and antiasthmatics
12. Herbs for improving appetite and digestion and removing food stagnation
13. Herbs for regulating Qi
14. Herbs for promoting circulation and removing blood stasis
15. Homostatic herbs
16. Tonics herbs
17. Herbs used as Astringents
18. Herbs used as Anthelmintics

Appendix Two summarises lists of commonly used Chinese medicinal herbs classified according to pharmacological actions. They are grouped into 16 categories.

A   Herbs for cardiovascular system (subdivided into 6 groups)
B   Herbs for respiratory system (subdivided into 3 groups)
C   Herbs for alimentary system (subdivided into 3 groups)
D   Herbs for the nervous system (subdivided into 6 groups)
E   Herbs for the genito-urinary system (subdivided into 2 groups)
F   Herbs used as tonics
G   Anti-inflammatory herbs
H   Antidiabetic herbs
I   Antibacterial herbs
J   Antiviral herbs
K   Antimycotic herbs

L Antimalarial herbs
M Antiamoebial herbs
N Antitrichomonial herbs
O Anticarcinogenic herbs
P Photosensitizer herbs

Appendix Three describes the lists of commonly used prescription formulae as ready-made Chinese herbal medicinal products. The majorities are well-known prescription products that are recorded in the Official Chinese Pharmacopoeia. Some local TCM practitioners have introduced some in the local market for use, as their philosophy was that people in the West might be more sensitive to CHM products. However very little published work has been available to substantiate this finding. These are different from the ones recognised and documented in the East. Those examples in the lists marked with asterisk are the products concerned. There are 101 examples quoted for reference. The major difficulties that these products facing are the quality assurance issues. These products do not fall into the medicinal category for regulation purposes in the most of the countries in the West. Apart from safety and efficacy variation in qualities of these imported products have been main concerns of the authorities. While these ready-made CHM products are convenient for use some TCM practitioners would like to have crude herbs available for their adjustment of number of herbs as judged from the patient's response during the course of treatment. Therefore the availability of guaranteed quality of crude CHM herbs is also essential.

APPENDIX 1: LISTS OF COMMONLY USED CHINESE MEDICINAL HERBS CLASSIFIED ACCORDING TO TRADITIONAL CHINESE MEDICINE ACTIONS (中药分类)

1. *Diaphoretics or Herbs for Treating Exterior Syndromes*   解表药
   (1) *Diaphoretics with pungent and warm properties*   辛温解表药
      Bai Zhi (Radix Angelicae Dahuricae)   白芷
      Fang Feng (Radix Ledebouriellae)   防风
      Gui Zhi (Ramulus Cinnamomi)   桂枝
      Jing Jie (Herba Schizonepetae)   荆芥
      Ma Huang (Herbs Ephedrae)   麻黄
      Qiang Huo (Rhizoma Seu Radix Notopterygii)   羌活
      Sheng Jiang (Rhizoma Zingiberis Recens)   生姜
      Su Ye (Folium Perillae)   苏叶
      Xin Yi (Flos Magnoliae)   辛夷
      Xi Xin (Herba Asari)   细辛
   (2) *Diaphoretics with pungent and cold properties*   辛凉解表药
      Bo He (Herba Menthae)   薄荷
      Chai Hu (Radix Bupleuri)   柴胡
      Dan Dou Chi (Semen Sojae Praeparatum)   淡豆豉
      Fu Ping (Herba Spirodelae)   浮萍
      Ge Gen (Radix Pueraeiae)   葛根
      Ju Hua (Flos Chrysanthemi)   菊花
      Man Jing Zi (Fructus Viticis)   蔓荆子
      Niu Bang Zi (Fructus Arctii)   牛蒡子
      Sang Ye (Folium Mori)   桑叶
      Sheng Ma (Rhizoma Cimicifugae)   开麻
2. *Heat-clearing Herbs*   清热药
   (1) *Heat-clearing and fire purging herbs*   清热泻火药
      Dan Zhu Ye (Folium Lophatheri)   淡竹叶
      Lu Gen (Rhizoma Phragmitis)   芦根
      Shi Gao (Gypsum Fibrosum)   石膏
      Tian Hua Fen (Radix Trichosanthis)   天花粉
      Zhi Mu (Rhizoma Anemarrhenae)   知母
      Zhi Zi (Fructus Gardeniae)   栀子
   (2) *Heat-clearing and detoxicating herbs*   清热解毒药
      Bai Hua She She Cao (Herba Hedyotis Diffusae)   白花蛇舌草
      Bai Jiang Cao (Herba Patriniae)   败酱草
      Bai Tou Weng (Radix Pulsatillae)   白头翁
      Bai Zhi Lian (Herba Scutellariae Barbatae)   半枝莲
      Chong Lou (Rhizoma Paridis)   重楼

    Jin Yin Hua (Flos Lonicerae) 金银花
    Lian Qiao (Fructus Forsythiae) 连翘
    Long Kui (Solanom Nigrum) 龙葵
    Ma Chi Xian (Herba Portulacae) 马齿苋
    Pu Gong Ying (Herba Taraxaci) 蒲公英
    Ren Dong Teng (Caulis Lonicerae) 忍冬藤
    Tu Fu Ling (Rhizoma Smilacis Galbrae) 土茯苓
    Wei Ling Cai (Herba Potentillae Chinensis) 委陵菜
    Yu Xing Cao (Herba Houttuyniae) 鱼腥草
    Zi Hua Di Ding (Herba Violae) 紫花地丁

(3) *Heat clearing and blood cooling herbs* 清热凉血药
    Chi Shao (Radix Paeoniae Rubra) 赤芍
    Da Qing Ye (Folium Isatidis) 大青叶
    Dan Pi (Cortex Moutan Radicis) 丹皮
    Mao Gen (Rhizoma Imperatae) 茅根
    Sheng Di Huang (Radix Rehmanniae) 生地黄
    Shui Niu Jiao (Cornu Bubalus) 水牛角
    Xuan Shen (Radix Scrophulariae) 玄参
    Zi Cao (Radix Arnebiae Seu Lithospermi) 紫草

(4) *Heat-clearing and dampness-drying* 清热燥湿药
    Bai Xian Pi (Cortex Dictamni Radicis) 白鲜皮
    Huang Bo (Cortex Phellodendri) 黄柏
    Huang Lian (Rhizoma Coptidis) 黄连
    Huang Qin (Radix Scutellariae) 黄芩
    Ku Shen (Radix Sophorae Flavescentis) 苦参
    Long Dan Cao (Radix Gentianae) 龙胆草
    Ming Fan (Alumen) 明矾
    Qin Pi (Cortex Fraxini) 秦皮

(5) *Herbs for heat-clearing from the liver to treat the eye diseases* 清肝明目药
    Mi Meng Hua (Flos Buddlejae) 密蒙花
    Xia Ku Cao (Spica Purnellae) 夏枯草

(6) *Herbs for clearing xu heat* 清虚热药
    Di Gu Pi (Cortex Lycii Radicis) 地骨皮
    Qing Hao (Herba Artemisiae Annuae) 青蒿

3. *Purgative Herbs* 泻下药
(1) *Purgative* 攻下药
    Da Huang (Radix Et Rhizoma Rhei) 大黄
    Fan Xie Ye (Folium Sennae) 番泻叶
    Mang Xiao (Natrii Sulfas) 芒硝
(2) *Laxative* 润下药
    Huo Ma Ren (Fructus Cannabis) 火麻仁
    Yu Li Ren (Semen Pruni) 郁李仁

4. *Aromatic Herbs for Resolving Dampness* 芳香化湿药
    Cang Zhu (Rhizoma Atractylodis) 苍术

Dou Kou (Fructus Amomi Rotundus) 豆蔻

Hou Po (Cortex Magnoliae Officinalis) 厚朴

Huo Xiang (Herba Pogostemomis) 藿香

Sha Ren (Fructus Amomi) 砂仁

5. *Herbs for Inducing Diuresis and Excreting Dampness* 利水渗湿药

Bi Xie (Rhizoma Dioscoreae Hypoglaucae) 萆薢

Bian Xu (Herba Polygoni Avicularis) 萹蓄

Che Qian Cao (Herba Plantaginis) 车前草

Che Qian Zi (Semen Plantaginis) 车前子

Di Fu Zi (Fructus Kochiae) 地肤子

Fu Ling (Poria) 茯苓

Hu Zhang (Rhizoma Polygoni Cuspidati) 虎杖

Hua Shi (Talcum) 滑石

Jin Qian Cao (Herba Lysimachiae) 金钱草

Mu Tong (Caulis Akebiae) 木通

Qu Mai (Herba Dianthi) 瞿麦

Tong Cao (Medulla Tetrapanacis) 通草

Yi Ren (Semen Coicis) 薏仁

Yin Chen (Herba Artemisiac Scopariae) 茵陈

Yu Mi Xu (Stigma Maydis) 玉米须

Ze Xie (Rhizoma Alismatis) 泽泻

Zhu Ling (Polyporus Umbellatus) 猪苓

6. *Antirheumatics (Herbs for Expelling Wind and Dampness)* 祛风湿药

Cang Er Zi (Fructus Xanthii) 苍耳子

Du Huo (Radix Angelicae Pubescentis) 独活

Hai Feng Teng (Caulis Piperis Futokadsurae) 海风藤

Mu Gua (Fructus Chaenomelis) 木瓜

Qin Jiao (Radix Gentianae Macrophyllae) 秦艽

Sang Ji Sheng (Ramulus Taxilli) 桑寄生

Sang Zhi (Ramulus Mori) 桑枝

Shen Jin Cao (Herba Lycopodii) 伸筋草

Wei Ling Xian (Radix Clematidis) 威灵仙

Wu Jia Pi (Cortex Acanthopanaci Radicis) 五加皮

Xi Qian Cao (Herba Siegesbeckiae) 豨莶草

7. *Interior Warming Herbs* 温里药

Ding Xiang (Flos Caryophlli) 丁香

Fu Zi (Radix Aconiti Praeparata) 附子

Gan Cao (Rhizoma Zingiberis) 干姜

Hua Jiao (Pericarpium Zanthoxyli) 花椒

Rou Gui (Cortex Cinnamomi) 肉桂

Wu Zhu Yu (Fructus Evodiae) 吴茱萸

8. *Herbs for Inducing Resusscitation* 开窍药

Shi Chang Pu (Rhixoma Acori Gramimei) 石菖蒲

9. *Sedatives and Tranquilizers Herbs* 安神药

(1) *Tranquilizers* 重镇安神药

Ci Shi (Magnetitum)   磁石
Long Gu (Os Draconis)   龙骨
Mu Li (Concha Ostreae)   牡蛎
Zhen Zhu (Margarita)   珍珠
Zhen Zhu Mu (Concha Margaritifera Usta)   珍珠母

(2) *Sedatives*   养心安神药
Bai Zi Ren (Semen Biotae)   柏子仁
He Huan Pi (Cortex Albizziae)   合欢皮
Suan Zao Ren (Semen Ziziphi Spinosae)   酸枣仁
Ye Jiao Teng (Caulis Polygoni Multiflori)   夜交藤
Yuan Zhi (Radix Polygalae)   远志

10. *Herbs for Calming the Liver to Check Endogenous Wind*   平肝息风药
Dai Zhe Shi (Haematitum)   代赭石
Gou Teng (Ramulus Uncariae Cum Uncis)   钩藤
Ji Li (Fructus Tribuli)   蒺藜
Shi Jue Ming (Concha Haliotidis)   石决明
Tian Ma (Rhizoma Gastrodiae)   天麻

11. *Expectorants, Antitussives and Antiasthmatics*   化痰止咳药
(1) *Herbs for resolving cold phlegm*   温化寒痰药
Ban Xia (Rhizoma Pinelliae)   半夏
Fu Zi (Rhizoma Typhonii)   附子
Jie Geng (Radix Platycodi)   桔梗
Tian Nan Xing (Rhizoma Arisaematis)   天南星
Xuan Fu Hua (Flos Inulae)   旋覆花
(2) *Herbs for resolving heat phlegm*   清化热痰药
Chuan Bei Mu (Bulbus Fritillariae Cirrhosae)   川贝母
Er Cha (Catechu)   儿茶
Fu Hai Shi (Pumex)   浮海石
Gua Lou (Fructus Trichosanthis)   瓜蒌
Ge Qiao (Concha Meretrigis Seu Cyclinae)   蛤壳
Hai Zao (Sargassum)   海藻
Kun Bo (Thallus Eckloniae)   昆布
Qian Hu (Radix Peucedani)   前胡
Wa Leng Zi (Concha Arcae)   瓦楞子
Zhe Bei Mu (Bulbus Fritillariae Thunbergii)   浙贝母
Zhu Ru (Caulis Bambusae In Taenian)   竹茹
(3) *Herbs for resolving cough and asthma*   止咳平喘药
Bai Bu (Radix Stemonae)   百部
Kuan Dong Hua (Flos Farfarae)   款冬花
Pi Pa Ye (Folium Eriobotryae)   枇杷叶
Xing Ren (Semen Armeniacae Amarum)   杏仁
Zi Yuan (Radix Asteris)   紫苑

12. *Herbs for Improving Appetite and Digestion and*   消导药
Removing Food Stagnation
Gu Ya (Fructus Oryzae Sativae Germinatus)   谷芽

Ji Nei Jin (Endothelium Corneum Gigeriae Galli) 鸡内金
Lai Fu Zi (Semen Raphani) 莱服子
Mai Ya (Fructus Hordei Germinatus) 麦芽
Shan Zha (Fructus Crataegi) 山楂
Shen Qu (Massa Medicata Fermantata) 神曲

13. *Herbs for Regulating Qi* 理气药
Chen Pi (Pericarpium Citri Reticulatae) 陈皮
Da Fu Pi (Pericarpium Arecae) 大腹皮
Mei Gui Hua (Rose) 玫瑰花
Mu Xiang (Radix Aucklandiae) 木香
Qing Pi (Pericarpium Citri Reticulatae Viride) 青皮
Wu Yao (Radix Linderae) 乌药
Xiang Fu (Rhizoma Cyperi) 香附
Zhi Shi (Fructus Aurantii Immaturus) 枳实
Zhi Qiao (Fructus Aurantii) 枳壳

14. *Herbs for Promoting Circulation and Removing Blood Stasis* 活血祛瘀药
Chuan Xiong (Rhizoma Ligustici Chuan Xiong) 川芎
Dan Shen (Radix Salviae Miltiorrhizae) 丹参
Hong Hua (Flos Carthami) 红花
Ji Xue Teng (Caulis Spatholobi) 鸡血藤
Ma Bian Cao (Herba Verbenae) 马鞭草
Mao Dong Qing (Radix Ilicis Pubescentis) 毛冬青
Niu Xi (Radix Achyranthis Bidentatae) 牛膝
Tao Ren (Semen Persicae) 桃仁
Wang Bu Liu Xing (Semen Vaccariae) 王不留行
Yuan Hu (Rhizoma Corydalis) 元胡
Yi Mu Cao (Herba Leonuri) 益母草
Yu Jin (Radix Curcumae) 郁金
Ze Lan (Herba Lycopi) 泽兰
Zi Ran Tong (Pyritum) 自然铜

15. *Hemostatics Herbs* 止血药
Da Ji (Radix Cirsii Japonici) 大蓟
Di Yu (Radix Sanguisorbae) 地榆
Huai Hua (Flos Sophorae) 槐花
Huai Jiao (Fructus Sophorae) 槐角
Pu Huang (Pollen Typhae) 蒲黄
San Qi (Radix Notoginseng) 三七
Xian He Cao (Herba Agrimoniae) 仙鹤草
Xiao Ji (Herba Cephalanoploris) 小蓟

16. *Tonics* 补益药
(1) *Herbs for Reinforcing Qi*
Bai Zhu (Rhizoma Atractylodis Macrocephalae) 白术
Bian Dou (Semen Dolichoris Album) 扁豆
Da Zao (Fructus Ziziphi Jujubae) 大枣
Dang Shen (Radix Codonopsis Pilosulae) 党参

Gan Cao (Radix Glycyrrhizae) 甘草
Hai Er Shen (Radix Pseudostellariae) 孩儿参
Huang Jing (Rhizoma Polygonati) 黄精
Huang Qi (Radix Astragali Seu Hedysari) 黄芪
Ren Shen (Radix Ginseng) 人参
Shan Yao (Rhizoma Dioscoreae) 山药
Xi Yang Shen (Radix Panacis Quinquefolii) 西洋参

(2) *Herbs for Tonifying Yang* 助阳药
Ba Ji Tian (Radix Morindae Officinalis) 巴戟天
Bu Gu Zhi (Fructus Psoraleae) 补骨脂
Du Zhong (Cortex Eucommiae) 杜仲
Ge Jie (Gecko) 蛤蚧
Gou Ji (Rhizoma Cibotii) 狗脊
Gu Sui Bu (Rhizoma Drynariae) 骨碎补
Hai Ma (Hippocampus) 海马
Lu Jiao Jiao (Colla Cornus Cervi) 鹿角胶
Lu Jiao Shuang (Cornu Cervi Degelatinatum) 鹿角霜
Rou Cong Rong (Herba Cistanches) 肉苁蓉
She Chuang Zi (Fructus Cnidii) 蛇床子
Tu Si Zi (Semen Cuscutae) 菟丝子
Xian Mao (Rhizoma Curculiginis) 仙茅
Xu Duan (Radix Dipsaci) 续断
Yi Zhi Ren (Fructus Alpiniae Oxyphyllae) 益智仁
Yin Yang Huo (Herba Epimedii) 淫羊藿

(3) *Herbs for Nourishing the Blood* 养血药
Bai Shao (Radix Paeoniae Alba) 白芍
Dang Gui (Radix Angelicae Sinensis) 当归
E Jiao (Colla Corii Asini) 阿胶
Long Yan Rou (Arillus Longan) 龙眼肉
Sang Shen (Fructus Mori) 桑椹
Shou Wu (Radix Polygori Multiflori) 首乌
Shu Di (Radix Rehmanniae Praeparata) 熟地

(4) *Herbs for Nourishing Yin* 滋阴药
Bai He (Bulbus Lilii) 百合
Gui Ban (Plastrum Testudinis) 龟板
Han Lian Cao (Herba Ecliptae) 旱莲草
Mai Dong (Radix Ophiopogonis) 麦冬
Nu Zhen Zi (Fructus Liqustri Lucidi) 女贞子
Qi Zi (Fructus Lycii) 杞子
Sha Shen (Radix Glenhiae) 沙参
Shi Hu (Herba Dendrobii) 石斛
Tian Dong (Radix Asparagi) 天冬
Yu Zhu (Rhizoma Polygonati Odorati) 玉竹

17. *Astringents* 固涩药
Bai Guo (Semen Ginkgo) 白果

Chi Shi Zhi (Halloysitum Rubrum)	赤石脂
Hai Piao Xiao (Os Sepellae Seu Sepiae)	海螵蛸
Ke Zi (Fructus Chebulae)	诃子
Lian Zi (Semen Nelumbinis)	莲子
Ming Fan (Alumen)	明矾
Qian Shi (Semen Euryales)	芡实
Sang Piao Xiao (Ootheca Mantidis)	桑螵蛸
Shan Zhu Yu (Fructus Corni)	山茱萸
Wu Bei Zi (Galla Chinensis)	五倍子
Wu Mei (Fructus Mume)	乌梅
Wu Wei Zi (Fructus Schisandrae)	五味子

18. *Anthelmintics*   驱虫药

Bing Lang (Semen Arecae)	槟榔

APPENDIX 2: LISTS OF COMMONLY USED CHINESE MEDICINAL HERBS CLASSIFIED ACCORDING TO PHARMACOLOGICAL ACTIONS (药理作用分类)

A. *Cardiovascular System*   心血管系统

(1)   *Antihypertensive Herbs:*   降血压药

Bai Zhu (Rhizoma Atractylodis Macrocephalae)	白术
Chuan Bei Mu (Bulbus Fritillariae Cirrhosae)	川贝母
Chuan Xiong (Rhizoma Ligustici Chuan Xiong)	川芎
Da Huang (Radix Et Rhizoma Rhei)	大黄
Dan Pi (Cortex Moutan Radicis)	丹皮
Dan Shen (Radix Salviae Miltiorrhizae)	丹参
Dang Gui (Radix Angelicae Sinensis)	当归
Di Gu Pi (Cortex Lycii Radicis)	地骨皮
Du Huo (Radix Angelicae Pubescentis)	独活
Du Zhong (Cortex Eucommiae)	杜仲
Ge Gen (Radix Pueraeiae)	葛根
Gou Teng (Ramulus Uncariae Cum Uncis)	钩藤
Hou Po (Cortex Magnoliae Officinalis)	厚朴
Hu Zhang (Rhizoma Polygoni Cuspidati)	虎杖
Huang Bo (Cortex Phellodendri)	黄柏
Huang Jing (Rhizoma Polygonati)	黄精
Huang Lian (Rhizoma Coptidis)	黄连
Huang Qi (Radix Astragali Seu Hedysari)	黄芪
Huang Qin (Radix Scutellariae)	黄芩

Jie Geng (Radix Platycodi) 桔梗
Jian Qian Cao (Herba Lysimachiae) 金钱草
Ku Shen (Radix Sophorae Flavescentis) 苦参
Lai Fu Zi (Semen Raphani) 莱菔子
Long Dan Cao (Radix Gentianae) 龙胆草
Long Kui (Solanom Nigrum) 龙葵
Mao Dong Qing (Radix Ilicis Pubescentis) 毛冬青
Mu Tong (Caulis Akebiae) 木通
Mu Xiang (Radix Aucklandiae) 木香
Niu Xi (Radix Achyranthis Bidentatae) 牛膝
Pu Huang (Pollen Typhae) 蒲黄
Qin Jiao (Radix Gentianae Macrophyllae) 秦艽
Qing Hao (Herba Artemisiae Annuae) 青蒿
Qu Mai (Herba Dianthi) 瞿麦
Ren Shen (Radix Ginseng) 人参
Rou Gui (Cortex Cinnamomi) 肉桂
San Qi (Radix Notoginseng) 三七
Sang Ji Sheng (Ramulus Taxilli) 桑寄生
Shan Zha (Fructus Crataegi) 山楂
Sheng Ma (Rhizoma Cimicifugae) 升麻
Suan Zho Ren (Semen Ziziphi Spinosae) 酸枣仁
Wu Wei Zi (Fructus Schisandrae) 五味子
Wu Zhu Yu (Fructus Evodiae) 吴茱萸
Xi Xian Cao (Herba Siegesbeckiae) 豨莶草
Xi Xin (Herba Asari) 细辛
Xia Ku Cao (Spica Prunellae) 夏枯草
Xiang Fu (Rhizoma Cyperi) 香附
Xin Yi (Flos Magnoliae) 辛夷
Xing Ren (Semen Armeniacae Amarum) 杏仁
Xuan Shen (Radix Scrophulariae) 玄参
Yin Chen (Herba Artemisiae Scopariae) 茵陈
Yin Yang Huo (Herba Epimedii) 淫羊藿
Yu Mi Xu (Stigma Maydis) 玉米须
Yuan Hu (Rhizoma Corydalis) 元胡
Ze Xie (Rhizoma Alismatis) 泽泻
Zhe Bei Mu (Bulbus Frutillariae Thunbergii) 浙贝母
Zhi Zi (Fructus Gardeniae) 栀子
(2) *Cardiotonic Herbs* 强心药
Bu Gu Zhi (Fructus Psoraleae) 补骨脂
Chen Pi (Pericarpium Citri Retuculatae) 陈皮
Chuan Xiong (Rhizoma Ligustici Chuan Xiong) 川芎
Du Zhong (Cortex Eucommiae) 杜仲
Fu Ling (Poria) 茯苓
Fu Zi (Radix Aconiti Praeparata) 附子
Lian Qiao (Fructus Forsythiae) 连翘

Ling Zhi (Gaboderma Lucidum)　　　　　　　　灵芝
Long Kui (Solanom Nigrum)　　　　　　　　　　龙葵
Mu Tong (Caulis Akebiae)　　　　　　　　　　木通
Niu Xi (Radix Achyranthis Bidentatae)　　　　牛膝
Nu Zhen Zi (Fructus Ligustri Lucidi)　　　　　女贞子
Ren Shen (Radix Genseng)　　　　　　　　　　人参
San Qi (Radix Notoginseng)　　　　　　　　　三七
Wu Wei Zi (Fructus Schisandrae)　　　　　　　五味子
Xi Xin (Herba Asari)　　　　　　　　　　　　细辛
Xian He Cao (Herba Agrimoniae)　　　　　　　仙鹤草
Xiang Fu (Rhizoma Cyperi)　　　　　　　　　　香附
Xuan Shen (Radix Scrophulariae)　　　　　　　玄参
Yu Zhu (Rhizoma Polygonati Odorati)　　　　　玉竹
Zhi Shi (Fructus Aurantii Immaturi)　　　　　枳实
Zhi Qiao (Fructus Aurantii)　　　　　　　　　枳壳

(3)　*Anticoagulant Herbs*　　　　　　　　　　抗凝血药
Bai Zhu (Rhizoma Atractylodis Macrocephalae)　白术
Chuan Xiong (Rhizoma Ligustici Chuan Xiong)　川芎
Dan Shen (Radix Salviae Miltiorrhizae)　　　　丹参
Dang Gui (Radix Angelicae Sinensis)　　　　　当归
Ge Gen (Radix Pueraeiae)　　　　　　　　　　葛根
Hong Hua (Flos Carthami)　　　　　　　　　　红花
Jin Qian Cao (Herba Lysimachiae)　　　　　　金钱草
Long Kui (Solanom Nigrum)　　　　　　　　　龙葵
Rou Gui (Cortex Cinnamomi)　　　　　　　　　肉桂
San Qi (Radix Notoginseng)　　　　　　　　　三七
Yin Chen (Herba Artemisiae Scopariae)　　　　茵陈

(4)　*Antiarrhythmic Herbs*　　　　　　　　　　抗心律不整药
Dang Gui (Radix Angelicae Sinensis)　　　　　当归
Huang Lian (Rhizoma Coptidis)　　　　　　　　黄连
Ku Shen (Radix Sophorae Flavescentis)　　　　苦参
Qing Hao (Herba Artemisiae Annuae)　　　　　青蒿
Tian Nan Xing (Rhizoma Arisaematis)　　　　　天南星
Yin Yang Huo (Herba Epimedii)　　　　　　　　淫羊藿

(5)　*Antianginal Herbs*　　　　　　　　　　　扩张冠状动脉药
Bu Gu Zhi (Fructus Psoraleae)　　　　　　　　补骨脂
Chen Pi (Pericarpium Citri Reticulatae)　　　陈皮
Chong Lou (Rhizoma Paridis)　　　　　　　　　重楼
Chuan Xiong (Rhizoma Ligustici Chuan Xiong)　川芎
Dan Shen (Radix Salviae Miltiorrhizae)　　　　丹参
Dang Gui (Radix Angelicae Sinensis)　　　　　当归
Ge Gen (Radix Pueraeiae)　　　　　　　　　　葛根
Hong Hua (Flos Carthami)　　　　　　　　　　红花
Hu Zhang (Rhizoma Polygoni Cuspidati)　　　　虎杖
Huang Lian (Rhizoma Coptidis)　　　　　　　　黄连

Huang Jing (Rhizoma Polygonati) 黄精
Huang Qi (Radix Astragali Seu Hedysari) 黄芪
Jin Qian Cao (Herba Lysimachiae) 金钱草
Ju Hua (Flos Carysanthemi) 菊花
Ling Zhi (Gaboderma Lucidum) 灵芝
Nu Zhen Zi (Fructus Ligustri Lucidi) 女贞子
Pu Huang (Pollen Typhae) 蒲黄
Qian Hu (Radix Peucedani) 前胡
Rou Gui (Cortex Cinnamomi) 肉桂
San Qi (Radix Notoginseng) 三七
Sang Ji Sheng (Ramulus Taxilli) 桑寄生
Shan Zha (Fructus Cartaegi) 山楂
Sheng Di Huang (Radix Rehmanniae) 生地黄
Shu Di (Radix Rehmanniae Praeparata) 熟地
Tian Ma (Rhizoma Gastrodiae) 天麻
Xi Xin (Herba Asari) 细辛
Yi Mu Cao (Herba Leonuri) 益母草
Yin Chen (Herba Artemisiae Scopariae) 茵陈
Yin Yang Huo (Herba Epimedii) 淫羊藿
Yuan Hu (Rhizoma Corydalis) 元胡
Zhe Bei Mu (Bulbus Fritillariae Thunbergii) 浙贝母
Ze Xie (Rhiaoma Alismatis) 泽泻

(6) *Antihypercholesterolemic Herbs* 降血脂药
Chai Hu (Radix Bupleuri) 柴胡
Chen Pi (Pericarpium Citri Reticulatae) 陈皮
Da Huang (Radix Et Rhizoma Rhei) 大黄
Dan Shen (Radix Salviae Miltiorrhizae) 丹参
Dang Gui (Radix Angelicae Sinensis) 当归
Di Gu Pi (Cortex Lycii Radicis) 地骨皮
Du Zhong (Cortex Eucommiae) 杜仲
Gan Cao (Radix Glycyrrhizae) 甘草
Hu Zhang (Rhizoma Polygoni Cuspidati) 虎杖
Huang Jing (Rhizoma Polygonati) 黄精
Jin Yin Hua (Flos Lonicerae) 金银花
Nu Zhen Zi (Fructus Liqustri Lucidi) 女贞子
Pu Huang (Pollen Typhae) 蒲黄
Qi Zi (Fructus Lycii) 杞子
Sang Ye (Folium Mori) 桑叶
Shan Zha (Fructus Crategi) 山楂
Shou Wu (Radix Polygori Multiflori) 首乌
Yin Chen (Herba Artemisiae Scopariae) 茵陈
Yin Yang Huo (Herba Epimedii) 淫羊藿
Ze Xie (Rhizoma Alismatis) 泽泻

B. *Respiratory System* 呼吸系统
(1) *Expectorants Herbs* 祛痰药

Bai Bu (Radix Stemonae) 百部
Bai Guo (Semen Ginkgo) 白果
Che Qian Cao (Herba Plantaginis) 车前草
Che Qian Zi (Semen Plantaginis) 车前子
Chen Pi (Pericarpium Citri Reticulatae) 陈皮
Chuan Bei Mu (Bulbus Fritillariae Cirrhosae) 川贝母
Gan Cao (Radix Glycyrrhizae) 甘草
Gua Lou (Fructus Trichosanthis) 瓜蒌
Jie Geng (Radix Platycodi) 桔梗
Ku Shen (Radix Sophorae Flavescentis) 苦参
Kuan Dong Hua (Flos Farfarae) 款冬花
Ling Zhi (Gaboderma Lucidum) 灵芝
Long Kui (Solanom Nigrum) 龙葵
Mao Dong Qing (Radix Illicis Puberseatis) 毛冬青
Qian Hu (Radix Peucedani) 前胡
Qin Pi (Cortex Fraxini) 秦皮
Qing Pi (Pericaprium Citri Reticulatae Viride) 青皮
Tian Nan Xing (Rhizoma Arisaematis) 天南星
Wu Wei Zi (Fructus Schisandrae) 五味子
Yin Yang Huo (Herba Epimedii) 淫羊藿
Yuan Zhi (Radix Polygalae) 远志

(2) *Antitussive Herbs* 镇咳药
Ban Xia (Rhizoma Pinelliae) 半夏
Bai Bu (Radix Stemonae) 百部
Cang Er Zi (Fructus Xanthii) 苍耳子
Chai Hu (Radix Bupleuri) 柴胡
Che Qian Cao (Herba Plantaginis) 车前草
Che Qian Zi (Semen Plantaginis) 车前子
Chuan Bei Mu (Bulbus Fritillariae Cirrhosae) 川贝母
Gan Cao (Radix Glycyrrhizae) 甘草
Gui Zhi (Ramulus Cinnamomi) 桂枝
Hu Zhang (Rhizoma Polygoni Cuspidati) 虎杖
Jie Geng (Radix Platycodi) 桔梗
Kuan Dong Hua (Flos Farfarae) 款冬花
Ling Zhi (Gaboderma Lucidum) 灵芝
Long Kui (Solanom Nigrum) 龙葵
Ma Huang (Herba Ephedrae) 麻黄
Mao Dong Qing (Radix Ilicis Pubesceatis) 毛冬青
Qin Pi (Cortex Fraxini) 秦皮
Wu Wei Zi (Fructus Schisandrae) 五味子
Xi Xin (Herba Asari) 细辛
Xing Ren (Semen Armeniacae Amarum) 杏仁
Xuan Fu Hua (Flos Inulae) 旋覆花
Yin Yang Huo (Herba Epimedii) 淫羊藿
Yu Xing Cao (Herba Houttuyniae) 鱼腥草

Zhe Bei Mu (Bulbus Fritillariae Thunbergii)   浙贝母

  (3)   *Antiasthmatic Herbs*   抗哮喘药

Bai Bu (Radix Stemonae)   百部

Chen Pi (Pericarpium Citri Reticulatae)   陈皮

Gui Zhi (Ramulus Cinnamom)   桂枝

Hu Zhang (Rhizoma Polygoni Cuspidati)   虎杖

Ku Shen (Radix Sophorae Flavescentis)   苦参

Kuan Dong Hua (Flos Farfarae)   款冬花

Ling Zhi (Gaboderma Lucidum)   灵芝

Long Kui (Solanom Nigrum)   龙葵

Qin Pi (Cortex Fraxini)   秦皮

Qing Pi (Pericaprium Citri Reticulatae Viride)   青皮

Xiang Fu (Rhizoma Cyperi)   香附

Xuan Fu Hua (Flos Inulae)   旋覆花

Yin Yang Huo (Herba Epimedii)   淫羊藿

C.   *Alimentary System*   消化系统

  (1)   *Herbs Promoting Digestion*   助消化药

Di Yu (Radix Sanguisorbae)   地榆

Gan Jiang (Rhizoma Zingiberis)   干姜

Gu Ya (Fructus Oryzae Sativae Germinatus)   谷芽

Ji Nei Jin (Endothelium Corneum Gigeriae Galli)   鸡内金

Jin Yin Hua (Flos Lonicerae)   金银花

Long Dan Cao (Radix Gentianae)   龙胆草

Mai Ya (Fructus Hordei Germinatus)   麦芽

Rou Gui (Cortex Cinnamomi)   肉桂

Shi Chang Pu (Rhizoma Acori Gramimei)   石菖蒲

Wu Yao (Radix Linderae)   乌药

  (2)   *Antacid and Antiulcer Herbs*   抗酸及抗溃疡药

Mu Li (Concha Ostreae)   牡蛎

Hai Piao Xiao (Os Sepiellae Seu Sepiae)   海螵蛸

Wa Leng Zi (Concha Arcae)   瓦楞子

  (3)   *Laxative Herbs*   致泻药

Da Huang (Radix Et Rhizoma Rhei)   大黄

Fan Xie Ye (Folium Sennae)   番泻叶

Gua Lou (Fructus Trichosanthis)   瓜蒌

Mang Xiao (Natrii Sulfas)   芒硝

Huo Ma Ren (Fructus Cannabis)   火麻仁

Yu Li Ren (Semen Pruni)   郁李仁

D.   *Nervous Systems*   神经系统

  (1)   *Hypnotic Herbs*   镇静催眠药

Bai Jiang Cao (Herba Patriniae)   败酱草

Chai Hu (Radix Bupleuri)   柴胡

Chuan Xiong (Rhizoma Ligustici Chuan Xiong)   川芎

Dan Shen (Radix Salviae Miltiorrhizae)   丹参

Dang Gui (Radix Angelicae Sinensis)   当归

Du Huo (Radix Angelicae Pubescentis)   独活
Du Zhong (Cortex Eucommiae)   杜仲
Fu Ling (Poria)   茯苓
Gou Teng (Ramulus Uncariae Cum Uncis)   钩藤
Gui Zhi (Ramulus Cinnamoni)   桂枝
Huang Lian (Rhizoma Coptidis)   黄连
Huang Qin (Radix Scutellariae)   黄芩
Hou Po (Cortex Magnoliae Officinalis)   厚朴
Ju Hua (Flos Chrysanthemi)   菊花
Ling Zhi (Gaboderma Lucidum)   灵芝
Long Dan Cao (Radix Gentianae)   龙胆草
Long Kui (Solamon Nigrum)   龙葵
Mu Tong (Caulis Akebiae)   木通
Qin Pi (Cortex Fraximi)   秦皮
Qin Jiao (Radix Gentianae Macrophyllae)   秦艽
Ren Shen (Radix Ginseng)   人参
Shan Zha (Fructus Crataegi)   山楂
Sheng Ma (Rhizoma Cimicifugae)   升麻
Shi Chang Pu (Rhizoma Acori Gramimei)   石菖蒲
Shu Di (Radix Rehmanniae Praeparata)   熟地
Shui Niu Jiao (Cornu Bubalus)   水牛角
Suan Zao Ren (Semen Ziziphi Spinosae)   酸枣仁
Tian Ma (Rhizoma Gastrodiae)   天麻
Tian Nan Xing (Rhizoma Arisaematis)   天南星
Xi Xin (Herba Asari)   细辛
Xiang Fu (Rhizoma Cyperi)   香附
Xuan Shen (Radix Scrophulariae)   玄参
Yi Ren (Semen Coicis)   薏仁
Yuan Hu (Rhizoma Corydalis)   元胡
Zhi Zi (Fructus Gardeniae)   栀子

(2) *Sedative Herbs*   安静药
Ren Shen (Radix Ginseng)   人参
Shi Chang Pu (Rhizoma Acori Gramimci)   石菖蒲
Suan Zao Ren (Semen Ziziphi Spinosae)   酸枣仁
Yuan Hu (Rhizoma Corydalis)   元胡

(3) *Anticonvulsive Herbs*   抗惊药
Dan Pi (Cortex Moutan Radicis)   丹皮
Fang Feng (Radix Ledebouriellae)   防风
Gan Cao (Radix Glycyrrhizae)   甘草
Gou Teng (Ramulus Uncariae Cum Uncis)   钩藤
Gui Zhi (Ramulus Cinnamomi)   桂枝
Long Dan Cao (Radix Gentianae)   龙胆草
Mu Tong (Caulis Akebiae)   木通
Qin Pi (Cortex Fraxini)   秦皮
Ren Shen (Radix Ginseng)   人参

Sheng Ma (Rhizoma Cimicifugae) 升麻
Shi Chang Pu (Rhizoma Acori Gramimei) 石菖蒲
Shui Niu Jiao (Cornu Bubalus) 水牛角
Suan Zao Ren (Semen Ziziphi Spinosae) 酸枣仁
Tian Nan Xing (Rhizoma Arisaematis) 天南星
Xuan Shen (Radix Scrophulariae) 玄参
Yuan Zhi (Radix Polygalae) 远志

(4) *Analgesic Herbs* 镇痛药
Dan Pi (Cortex Moutan Radicis) 丹皮
Dan Shen (Radix Salviae Miltiorrhizae) 丹参
Dang Gui (Radix Angelicae Sinensis) 当归
Du Huo (Radix Angelicae Pubescentis) 独活
Du Zhong (Cortex Eucommiae) 杜仲
Fang Feng (Radix Ledebouriellae) 防风
Gan Cao (Radix Glycyrrhizae) 甘草
Gan Jiang (Rhizoma Zingiberis) 干姜
Gui Zhi (Ramulus Cinnamomi) 桂枝
Ling Zhi (Gaboderma Lucidum) 灵芝
Long Kui (Solamon Nigrum) 龙葵
Mu Tong (Caulis Akebiae) 木通
Niu Xi (Radix Achyranthis Bidentatae) 牛膝
Qing Hao (Herba Artemisiae Annuae) 青蒿
Qin Jiao (Radix Gentianae Macrophyllae) 秦艽
Ren Shen (Radix Ginseng) 人参
Sheng Ma (Rhizoma Cimicifugae) 升麻
Suan Zao Ren (Semen Ziziphi Spinosae) 酸枣仁
Tian Nan Xing (Rhizoma Arisaematis) 天南星
Wu Zhu Yu (Fructus Evocdiae) 吴茱萸
Xi Xin (Herba Asari) 细辛
Xiang Fu (Rhizoma Cyperi) 香附
Xian He Cao (Herba Agrimoniae) 仙鹤草
Yi Ren (Semen Coicis) 薏仁
Zhi Zi (Fructus Gardeniae) 栀子

(5) *Antipyretic Herbs* 退热药
Bo He (Herba Menthae) 薄荷
Chai Hu (Radix Bupleuri) 柴胡
Da Qing Ye (Folium Isatidis) 大青叶
Dan Pi (Cortex Moutan Radicis) 丹皮
Dan Shen (Radix Salviae Miltiorrhizae) 丹参
Dan Zhu Ye (Folium Lophatheri) 淡竹叶
Di Gu Pi (Cortex Lycii Radicis) 地骨皮
Gan Cao (Radix Glycyrrhizae) 甘草
Ge Gen (Radix Pueraeiac) 葛根
Gui Zhi (Ramulus Cinnamomi) 桂枝
Huang Lian (Rhizoma Coptidis) 黄连

Huang Qin (Radix Scutellariae)　　黄芩
Jin Yin Hua (Flos Lonicerae)　　金银花
Jing Jie (Herba Schizonepetae)　　荆芥
Lian Qiao (Fructus Forysthiae)　　连翘
Long Kui (Solamon Nigrum)　　龙葵
Ma Huang (Herba Ephedrae)　　麻黄
Qin Jiao (Radix Gentianae Macrophyllae)　　秦艽
Qing Hao (Herba Artemisiae Annuae)　　青蒿
Sheng Ma (Rhizoma Cimicifugae)　　升麻
Shi Gao (Gypsum Fibrosum)　　石膏
Xi Xin (Herba Asari)　　细辛
Xiang Fu (Rhizoma Cyperi)　　香附
Xuan Shen (Radix Scrophulariae)　　玄参
Yi Ren (Semen Coicis)　　薏仁
Yin Chen (Herba Artemisiae Scopariae)　　茵陈
Zhi Mu (Rhizoma Anemarrhenae)　　知母

(6) *Central Stimulating Herbs*　　中枢兴奋药
Du Huo (Radix Angelicae Pubescentis)　　独活
Huang Lian (Rhizoma Coptidis)　　黄连
Jin Yin Hua (Flos Lonicerae)　　金银花
Kuan Dong Hua (Flos Farfarae)　　款冬花
Ma Huang (Herba Ephedrae)　　麻黄
Qin Jiao (Radix Gentianae Macrophyllae)　　秦艽
Ren Shen (Radis Ginseng)　　人参
Wu Wei Zi (Fructus Schisandrae)　　五味子
Wu Zhi Yu (Fructus Evodiae)　　吴茱萸
Xi Xin (Herba Asari)　　细辛

E. *Genitourinary System*　　泌尿系统
(1) *Diuretic Herbs*　　利尿药
Bai Zhu (Rhizoma Atractylodis Macrocephalae)　　白术
Che Qian Cao (Herba Plantaginis)　　车前草
Che Qian Zi (Semen Plantaginis)　　车前子
Cang Zhu (Rhizoma Atractylodis)　　苍术
Da Huang (Radix Et Rhizomz Rhei)　　大黄
Dan Zhu Ye (Herba Lophatheri)　　淡竹叶
Dang Gui (Radix Angelicae Sinensis)　　当归
Du Zhong (Cortex Eucommiae)　　杜仲
Fu Ling (Poria)　　茯苓
Gui Zhi (Ramulus Cinnamomi)　　桂枝
Huang Qi (Radix Astragali Seu Hedysari)　　黄芪
Huang Qin (Radix Scutellariae)　　黄芩
Jie Geng (Radix Platycodi)　　桔梗
Jin Qian Cao (Herba Lysimachiae)　　金钱草
Ku Shen (Radix Sophorae Flavescentis)　　苦参
Lian Qiao (Fructus Forsythiae)　　连翘

Ma Huang (Herba Ephedrae) 麻黄
Mao Gen (Rhizoma Imperatae) 茅根
Mu Tong (Caulis Akebiae) 木通
Qin Pi (Cortex Traxini) 秦皮
Qu Mai (Herba Dianthi) 瞿麦
San Qi (Radix Notoginseng) 三七
Sang Ji Sheng (Ramulus Taxilli) 桑寄生
Shu Di (Radix Rehmanniae Praeparata) 熟地
Yin Chen (Herba Artemisiae Scopariae) 茵陈
Yu Mi Xu (Stigma Maydis) 玉米须
Yu Xing Cao (Herba Houttuyniae) 鱼腥草
Ze Xie (Rhizoma Alismatis) 泽泻
Zhi Qiao (Fructus Aurantii) 枳壳
Zhu Ling (Polyporus Umbellatus) 猪苓

(2) *Herbs Affecting the Uterus* 作用于子宫药
Chuan Bei Mu (Bulbus Fritillariae Cirrhosae) 川贝母
Chuan Xiong (Rhizoma Ligustici Chuan Xiong) 川芎
Da Qing Ye (Folium Isatidis) 大青叶
Dang Gui (Radix Angelicae Sinensis) 当归
Di Gu Pi (Cortex Lycii Radicis) 地骨皮
Hong Hua (Flos Carthami) 红花
Huang Lian (Rhizoma Coptidis) 黄连
Jin Yin Hua (Flos Lonicerae) 金银花
Kuan Dong Hua (Flos Farfarae) 款冬花
Mu Tong (Caulis Akebiae) 木通
Niu Xi (Radix Achyranthis Bidentatae) 牛膝
Pu Huang (Pollen Typhae) 蒲黄
Qin Pi (Cortex Fraxini) 秦皮
San Qi (Radix Notoginseng) 三七
Wu Wei Zi (Fructus Schisandrae) 五味子
Wu Zhu Yu (Fructus Evodiae) 吴茱萸
Xia Ku Cao (Spica Prunellae) 夏枯草
Xiang Fu (Rhizoma Cyperi) 香附
Xin Yi (Flos Magnoliae) 辛夷
Yi Mu Cao (Herba Leonuri) 益母草
Yuan Zhi (Radix Polygalae) 远志
Zhe Bei Mu (Bulbus Fritillariae Thunbergii) 浙贝母

F. *Tonics Herbs* 补益药
Dang Gui (Radix Angelicae Sinensis) 当归
Dang Shen (Radix Codonopsis Pilosulae) 党参
E Jiao (Colla Corii Asini) 阿胶
Qi Zi (Fructus Lycii) 杞子
Ren Shen (Radix Ginseng) 人参

G. *Anti-inflammatory Herbs* 抗炎症药
Chai Hu (Radix Bupleuri) 柴胡

Che Qian Cao (Herba Plantaginis)　车前草
Da Qing Ye (Folium Isatidis)　大青叶
Dan Pi (Cortex Moutan Radicis)　丹皮
Dan Shen (Radix Salviae Miltiorrhizae)　丹参
Dang Gui (Radix Angelicae Sinensis)　当归
Du Huo (Radix Angelicae Pubescentis)　独活
Du Zhong (Cortex Eucommiae)　杜仲
Fang Feng (Radix Ledebouriellae)　防风
Fu Zi (Radix Aconiti Praeparata)　附子
Gan Cao (Radix Glycyrrhizae)　甘草
Gan Jiang (Rhizoma Zingiberis)　干姜
Ge Gen (Radix Pueraeiae)　葛根
Huang Qin (Radix Scutellariae)　黄芩
Jin Yin Hua (Flor Lonicerae)　金银花
Lai Fu Zi (Semen Raphani)　莱菔子
Lian Qiao (Fructus Forysthiae)　连翘
Long Dan Cao (Radix Gentianae)　龙胆草
Long Kui (Solanom Nigrum)　龙葵
Ma Huang (Herba Ephedrae)　麻黄
Mu Tong (Caulis Akebiae)　木通
Niu Xi (Radix Achyranthis Bidentatae)　牛膝
Pu Huang (Pollen Typhae)　蒲黄
Qin Jiao (Radix Gentianae Macrophyllae)　秦艽
Qin Pi (Cortex Fraxini)　秦皮
Ren Shen (Radix Ginseng)　人参
Sheng Ma (Herba Cimicifugae)　升麻
Shu Di (Radix Rehmanniae Praeparata)　熟地
Shui Niu Jiao (Cornu Bubalus)　水牛角
Xi Xiang Cao (Herba Seigesbeckiae)　豨莶草
Xi Xin (Herba Asari)　细辛
Xian He Cao (Herba Agrimoniae)　仙鹤草
Xiang Fu (Rhizoma Cyperi)　香附
Xuan Shen (Radix Scrophulariae)　玄参
Yu Xin Cao (Herba Houttuyniae)　鱼腥草
Yin Yang Huo (Herba Epimedii)　淫羊藿

II. Antidiabetic Herbs　降血糖药

Bai Zhu (Rhizoma Atractylodis Macroccphalae)　白术
Cang Er Zi (Fructus Xanthii)　苍耳子
Cang Zhu (Rhizoma Atractylodis)　苍术
Dan Shen (Radix Salviae Miltiorrhizae)　丹参
Di Gu Pi (Cortex Lycii Radicis)　地骨皮
Huang Jing (Rhizoma Pulygonati)　黄精
Jie Geng (Radix Platycodi)　桔梗
Mai Ya (Fructus Hordei Germinatus)　麦芽
Qi Zi (Fructus Lycii)　杞子

Sang Ye (Folium Mori)   桑叶
Shu Di (Radix Rehmanniae Praeparata)   熟地
Xian He Cao (Herba Agrimoniae)   仙鹤草
Xuan Shen (Radix Scrophulariae)   玄参
Yin Yang Huo (Herba Epimedii)   淫羊藿
Yu Mi Xu (Stigma Maydis)   玉米须
Yu Zhu (Rhizoma Polygonati Odorati)   玉竹
Ze Xie (Rhizoma Alismatis)   泽泻
Zhi Mu (Rhizoma Anemarrhenae)   知母

I. *Antibacterial Herbs*   抗细菌药

Bai Bu (Radix Stemonae)   百部
Bai Hua She She Cao (Herba Hedyotis Diffusae)   白花蛇舌草
Bai Jiang Cao (Herba Patriniae)   败酱草
Bai Tou Weng (Radix Pulsatillae)   白头翁
Bing Lang (Semen Arecae)   槟榔
Bo He (Herba Menthae)   薄荷
Bu Gu Zhi (Fructus Psoraleae)   补骨脂
Cang Er Zi (Fructus Xanthii)   苍耳子
Cang Zhu (Rhizoma Atractylodis)   苍术
Chai Hu (Radix Bupleuri)   柴胡
Chen Pi (Pericarpium Citri Reticulatae)   陈皮
Da Huang (Radix Et Rhizoma Rhei)   大黄
Da Qing Ye (Folium Isatidis)   大青叶
Dan Shen (Radix Salviae Miltiorrhizae)   丹参
Dan Pi (Cortex Moutan Radicis)   丹皮
Dan Zhu Ye (Folium Lophatheri)   淡竹叶
Dang Gui (Radix Angelicae Sinensis)   当归
Di Gu Pi (Cortex Lycii Radicis)   地骨皮
Di Yu (Radix Sanguisorbae)   地榆
Du Zhong (Cortex Eucommiae)   杜仲
Fang Feng (Radix Ledebouriellae)   防风
Gan Cao (Radix Glycyrrhizae)   甘草
Gua Lou (Fructus Trichosanthis)   瓜蒌
Gui Zhi (Ramulus Cinnamomi)   桂枝
Hou Po (Cortex Magnoliae Officinalis)   厚朴
Hu Zhang (Rhizoma Polygoni Cuspidati)   虎杖
Huang Bo (Cortex Phellodendri)   黄柏
Huang Jing (Rhizoma Pulygonati)   黄精
Huang Lian (Rhizoma Coptidis)   黄连
Huang Qi (Radix Astragali Seu Hedysari)   黄芪
Huang Qin (Radix Scutellariae)   黄芩
Jin Qian Cao (Herba Lysimachiae)   金钱草
Jin Yin Hua (Flos Lonincerae)   金银花
Ju Hua (Flos Chrysanthemi)   菊花
Ku Shen (Radix Sophorae flavescentis)   苦参

Lai Fu Zi (Semen Raphani) 莱菔子

Lian Qiao (Fructus Forysthiae) 连翘

Long Dan Cao (Radix Gentianae) 龙胆草

Long Kui (Solanom Nigrum) 龙葵

Ma Huang (Hereba Epaedrae) 麻黄

Mai Dong (Radix Ophiopogonis) 麦冬

Mao Dong Qing (Radix Ilicis Pubescentis) 毛冬青

Mao Gen (Rhizoma Imperatae) 茅根

Mu Tong (Caulis Akebiae) 木通

Nu Zhen Zi (Fructus Liqustri Lucidi) 女贞子

Pu Gong Ying (Herba Taraxaci) 蒲公英

Qian Hu (Radix Peucedani) 前胡

Qin Pi (Cortex Fraxini) 秦皮

Ren Shen (Radix Ginseng) 人参

Rou Gui (Cortex Cinnamomi) 肉桂

Sang Ye (Folium Mori) 桑叶

Sang Zhi (Ramulus Mori) 桑枝

Shan Zha (Fructus Crataegi) 山楂

Sheng Ma (Rhizoma Cimicifugae) 升麻

Shou Wu (Radix Polygori Multiflori) 首乌

Wu Mei (Fructus Mume) 乌梅

Wu Wei Zi (Fructus Schisandrae) 五味子

Wu Yao (Radix Linderae) 乌药

Wu Zhu Yu (Fructus Evodiae) 吴茱萸

Xi Xin (Herba Asari) 细辛

Xia Ku Cao (Spica Prunellae) 夏枯草

Xian He Cao (Herba Agrimoniae) 仙鹤草

Xiang Fu (Rhizoma Cyperi) 香附

Xin Yi (Flos Magnoliae) 辛夷

Xuan Fu Hua (Flos Inulae) 旋覆花

Xuan Shen (Radix Scrophulariae) 玄参

Yi Ren (Semen Coicis) 薏仁

Ying Yang Huo (Herba Epimedii) 淫羊藿

Yu Xing Cao (Herba Houttuyniae) 鱼腥草

Zhi Mu (Rhizoma Anemarrhenae) 知母

Zhi Zi (Fructus Gardeniae) 栀子

J.   Antiviral Herbs 抗病毒药

Bai Bu (Radix Stemonae) 百部

Bai Tou Weng (Radix Pulsatillae) 白头翁

Bing Lang (Semen Arecae) 槟榔

Bo He (Herba Menthae) 薄荷

Chai Hu (Radix Bupleuri) 柴胡

Da Huang (Radix Et Rhizoma Rhei) 大黄

Da Qing Ye (Folium Isatidis) 大青叶

Di Gu Pi (Cortex Lycii Radicis) 地骨皮

Di Yu (Radix Sanguisorbae)   地榆
Fang Feng (Radix Ledebouriellae)   防风
Gui Zhi (Ramulus Cinnamomi)   桂枝
Hou Po (Cortex Magnoliae Officinalis)   厚朴
Hu Zhang (Rhizoma Polygoni Cuspidati)   虎杖
Huang Bo (Cortex Phellodendri)   黄柏
Huang Jing (Rhizoma Pulygonati)   黄精
Huang Lian (Rhizoma Coptidis)   黄连
Huang Qin (Radix Scutellariae)   黄芩
Jin Yin Hua (Flos Lonicerae)   金银花
Ju Hua (Flos Chrysanthemi)   菊花
Lian Qiao (Fructus Forysthiae)   连翘
Ma Huang (Herba Epaedrae)   麻黄
Nu Zhen Zi (Fructus Liqustri Lucidi)   女贞子
Pu Gong Ying (Herba Tarazaci)   蒲公英
San Qi (Radix Notoginseng)   三七
Sang Ji Sheng (Ramulus Taxilli)   桑寄生
She Chuang Zi (Fructus Cnidii)   蛇床子
Xin Yi (Flos Magnoliae)   辛夷
Yin Chen (Herba Artemisiae Scopariae)   茵陈
Yin Yang Huo (Herba Epimedii)   淫羊藿
Yu Xing Cao (Herba Houttuyniae)   鱼腥草

K. *Antimycotic Herbs*   抗真菌药
Bai Bu (Radix Stemonae)   百部
Bai Tou Weng (Radix Pulsatillae)   白头翁
Bing Lang (Semen Arecae)   槟榔
Bu Gu Zhi (Fructus Psoraleae)   补骨脂
Cang Er Zi (Fructus Xanthii)   苍耳子
Che Qian Cao (Herba Plantaginis)   车前草
Chuan Bei Mu (Bulbus Fritillariae Cirrhosae)   川贝母
Da Huang (Radix Et Rhizoma Rhei)   大黄
Dan Pi (Cortex Moutan Radicis)   丹皮
Dan Shen (Radix Salviae Miltiorrhizae)   丹参
Fang Feng (Radix Ledebouriellae)   防风
Gua Lou (Fructus Trichosanthis)   瓜蒌
Gui Zhi (Ramulus Cinnamomi)   桂枝
Huang Bo (Cortex Phellodendri)   黄柏
Huang Jing (Rhizoma Pulygonati)   黄精
Huang Lian (Rhizoma Coptidis)   黄连
Jie Geng (Radix Platycodi)   桔梗
Ju Hua (Flos Chrysanthemi)   菊花
Ku Shen (Radix Sophorae Flavescentis)   苦参
Lai Fu Zi (Semen Raphani)   莱菔子
Lian Qiao (Fructus Forsythiae)   连翘
Long Kui (Solamon Nigrum)   龙葵

Mu Tong (Caulis Akebiae)	木通
Qian Jiao (Radix Gentianae Macrophyllae)	秦艽
Qing Hao (Herba Artemisiae Annuae)	青蒿
Rou Gui (Cortex Cinnamomi)	肉桂
San Qi (Radix Notoginseng)	三七
She Chuang Zi (Fructus Cnidii)	蛇床子
Sheng Ma (Rhizoma Cimicifugae)	升麻
Sheng Jiang (Rhizoma Zingiberis Recens)	生姜
Shi Chang Pu (Rhizoma Acori Gramimei)	石菖蒲
Shu Di (Radix Rehmanniae Praeparata)	熟地
Wei Ling Xian (Radix Clematidis)	威灵仙
Wu Mei (Fructus Mume)	乌梅
Wu Zhu Yu (Fructus Evodiae)	吴茱萸
Xiang Fu (Rhizoma Cyperi)	香附
Xin Yi (Flos Magnoliae)	辛夷
Xuan Shen (Radix Scrophulariae)	玄参
Yin Chen (Herba Artemisiae Capillaris)	茵陈
Yi Mu Cao (Herba Leonuri)	益母草
Jin Yin Hua (Flos Lonicerae)	金银花
Yu Xing Cao (Herba Houttuyniae)	鱼腥草
Zhi Mu (Rhizoma Anemarrhenae)	知母
Zhi Zi (Fructus Gardeniae)	栀子

L. *Antimalaria Herbs* — 抗疟疾药

Chai Hu (Radix Bupleuri)	柴胡
Long Dan Cao (Radix Gentianae)	龙胆草
Qing Hao (Herba Artemisiae Annuae)	青蒿

M. *Antiamebial Herbs* — 抗阿米巴药

Bai Tou Weng (Radix Pulsatillae)	白头翁
Da Huang (Radix Et Rhizoma Rhei)	大黄
Gan Cao (Radix Glycyrrhizae)	甘草
Ku Shen (Radix Sophorae Flavescentis)	苦参
She Chuang Zi (Fructus Cnidii)	蛇床子
Sheng Jiang (Rhizoma Zingiberis Recens)	生姜
Xian He Cao (Herba Agrimoniae)	仙鹤草

N. *Antitrichomonial Herbs* — 抗滴虫药

Bai Tou Weng (Radix Pulsatillae)	白头翁
Da Huang (Radix Et Rhizoma Rhei)	大黄
Gan Cao (Radix Glycyrrhizae)	甘草
Huang Bo (Cortex Phellodendri)	黄柏
Huang Lian (Rhizoma Coptidis)	黄连
Ku Shen (Radix Sophorae Flavescentis)	苦参
She Chuang Zi (Fructus Cnidii)	蛇床子
Sheng Jiang (Rhizoma Zingiberis Recens)	生姜
Xian He Cao (Herba Agrimoniae)	仙鹤草

O. Anticarcinogenic Herbs   抗肿瘤药
    Bai Hua She She Cao (Herba Hedyotis Diffusae)   白花蛇舌草
    Bai Jiang Cao (Herba Patriniae)   败酱草
    Bai Zhu (Rhizoma Atractylodis Macrocephalae)   白术
    Ban Xia (Rhizoma Pinelliae)   半夏
    Bo He (Herba Menthae)   薄荷
    Bu Gu Zhi (Fructus Psoraleae)   补骨脂
    Da Huang (Radix Et Rhizoma Rhei)   大黄
    Dan Shen (Radix Salviae Miltiorrhizae)   丹参
    Fu Ling (Poria)   茯苓
    Gan Cao (Radix Glychrrhizae)   甘草
    Gua Lou (Fructus Trichosanthis)   瓜蒌
    Huang Lian (Rhizoma Coptidis)   黄连
    Jin Yin Hua (Flos Lonicerae)   金银花
    Ku Shen (Radix Sophorae Flavescentis)   苦参
    Long Kui (Solamom Nigrum)   龙葵
    Nu Zhen Zi (Fructus Liqustri Lucidi)   女贞子
    Ren Shen (Radix Ginseng)   人参
    Shi Chang Pu (Rhizoma Acori Gramimei)   石菖蒲
    Sheng Ma (Rhizoma Cimicifugae)   升麻
    Tian Hua Fen (Radix Trichosanthis)   天花粉
    Tian Nan Xing (Rhizoma Arisaematis)   天南星
    We Mei (Fructus Mume)   乌梅
    Xia Ku Cao (Spica Purnellae)   夏枯草
    Xian He Cao (Herba Agrimoniae)   仙鹤草
    Xing Ren (Semen Armeniacae Amarum)   杏仁
    Yi Ren (Semen Coicis)   薏仁
    Yu Xing Cao (Herba Houttuyniae)   鱼腥草
    Zhu Ling (Polyporus Umbellatus)   猪苓
P. Photosensitizer Herbs   对光敏感药
    Bu Gu Zhi (Fructus Psoraleae)   补骨脂
    Du Huo (Radix Angelicae Pubescentis)   独活

APPENDIX 3: LISTS OF COMMONLY USED PRESCRIPTION FORMULAE AS READY MADE CHINESE HERBAL MEDICINAL PRODUCTS (中成药)

1. *Ba Zhen Tang*　　　　　　　　　　　　　　　　八珍汤
   Ren Shen (Radix Ginseng)　　　　　　　　　　　人参
   Bai Zhu (Rhizoma Atractylodis Macrocephalae)　　白术
   Fu Ling (Poria)　　　　　　　　　　　　　　　茯苓
   Gan Cao (Radix Glycyrrhizae)　　　　　　　　　甘草
   Shu Di Huang (Radix Rehmanniae Praeparata)　　熟地黄
   Dang Gui (Radix Angelica Sinensis)　　　　　　当归
   Bai Shao (Radix Paeoniae Alba)　　　　　　　　白芍
   Chuan Xiong (Rhizoma Chuanxiong)　　　　　　川芎

2. *Break into a Smile**　　　　　　　　　　　　　
   Chai Hu (Radix Bupleuri)　　　　　　　　　　　柴胡
   Bai Shao (Radix Paeoniae Alba)　　　　　　　　白芍
   Gan Cao (Radix Glycyrrhizae)　　　　　　　　　甘草
   Zhi Qiao (Fructus Aurantii)　　　　　　　　　　枳壳
   Chen Pi (Pericarpium Citrireticulatae)　　　　　陈皮
   Xiang Fu (Rhizoma Cyperi)　　　　　　　　　　香附
   Chuan Xiong (Rhizoma Chuanxiong)　　　　　　川芎
   Dan Shen (Radix Salviae Miltiorrhizae)　　　　　丹参
   Tai Zi Shen (Radix Pseudostellariae)　　　　　　太子参
   Yuan Hu (Rhizoma Corydalis)　　　　　　　　　元胡
   Suan Zao Ren (Smen Ziziphi Spinosae)　　　　　酸枣仁
   Fu Ling (Poria)　　　　　　　　　　　　　　　茯苓

3. *Bai Du San*　　　　　　　　　　　　　　　　败毒散
   Qiang Huo (Rhizoma Seu Radix Notopterygii)　　羌活
   Du Huo (Radix Angelicae Pubescens)　　　　　　独活
   Chai Hu (Radix Bupleuri)　　　　　　　　　　　柴胡
   Qian Hu (Radix Peucedani)　　　　　　　　　　前胡
   Chuan Xiong (Rhizoma Chuanxiong)　　　　　　川芎
   Dang Shen (Radix Codonopsis Pilosulae)　　　　党参
   Zhi Qiao (Fructus Aurantii)　　　　　　　　　　枳壳
   Fu Ling (Poria)　　　　　　　　　　　　　　　茯苓
   Jie Geng (Radix Platycodi)　　　　　　　　　　桔梗
   Gan Cao (Radix Glycyrrhizae)　　　　　　　　　甘草
   Bo He (Herba Menthae)　　　　　　　　　　　　薄荷
   Sheng Jiang (Rhizoma Zingiberis Recens)　　　　生姜

4. *Bai Hu Tang*   白虎汤
    Shi Gao (Gypsum Fibrosum)   石膏
    Zhi Mu (Rhizoma Anemarrhenae)   知母
    Gan Cao (Radix Glycyrrhizae)   甘草
    Rice   粳米

5. *Ban Xia Bai Zhu Tian Ma Tang*   半夏白术天麻汤
    Ban Xia (Rhizoma Pinelliae)   半夏
    Tian Ma (Rhizoma Gastrodiae)   天麻
    Bai Zhu (Rhizoma Atractylodis Macrocephalae)   白术
    Chen Pi (Pericarpium Citriretriculatae)   陈皮
    Gan Cao (Radix Glycyrrhizae)   甘草
    Sheng Jian (Rhizoma Zingberis Recens)   生姜
    Da Zao (Fructus Jujubae)   大枣

6. *Ban Xia Hou Po Tang*   半夏厚朴汤
    Ban Xia (Rhizoma Pinelliae)   半夏
    Hou Po (Cortex Magnoliae Officinalis)   厚朴
    Fu Ling (Poria)   茯苓
    Sheng Jiang (Rhizoma Zingiberis Recens)   生姜
    Su Ye (Folium Perillae)   苏叶

7. *Ban Xia Xie Xin Tang*   半夏泻心汤
    Ban Xia (Rhizoma Pinelliae)   半夏
    Gan Jiang (Rhizoma Zinguberis)   干姜
    Huang Qin (Radix Scutellariae)   黄岑
    Huang Lian (Rhizoma Coptidis)   黄连
    Ren Shen (Radix Ginseng)   人参
    Gan Cao (Radix Glycyrrhizae)   甘草
    Da Zao (Fructus Jujubae)   大枣

8. *Bend Bamboo**
    Dang Gui (Radix Angelica Sinensis)   当归
    Chuan Xiong (Rhizoma Chuanxiong)   川芎
    Shu Di Huang (Radix Rehmanniae Praeparata)   熟地黄
    Sang Ji Sheng (Herba Taxilli)   桑寄生
    Bai Shao (Radix Paeoniae Alba)   白芍
    Ju Hua (Flos Chrisanthemi)   菊花
    Tian Ma (Rhizoma Gastrodiae)   天麻
    Man Jing Zi (Fructus Viticis)   蔓荆子
    Ji Li (Fructus Tribuli)   蒺藜
    Fu Ling (Poria)   茯苓
    Qi Zi (Fructus Lycii)   杞子
    Gan Cao (Radix Glycyrrhizae)   甘草

9. *Bao He Wan* 保和丸
   Shan Zha (Fructus Crataegi) 山楂
   Shen Qu (Massa Fermentata Medicalis) 神曲
   Lai Fu Zi (Semen Raphani) 莱菔子
   Chen Pi (Pericarpium Citrireticulatae) 陈皮
   Ban Xia (Rhizoma Pinelliae) 半夏
   Fu Ling (Poria) 茯苓
   Lian Qiao (Fructus Forsythiae) 连翘

10. *Bi Xie Fen Qing Yin* 萆薢分清饮
    Bi Xie (Rhizoma Dioscoreae Hypoglaucae) 萆薢
    Yi Zhi Ren (Fructus Alpiniae Oxyphyllae) 益智仁
    Shi Chang Pu (Rhizoma Acori Tatarinowii) 石菖蒲
    Wu Yao (Radix Linderae) 乌药
    Fu Ling (Poria) 茯苓
    Gan Cao (Radix Glycyrrhizae) 甘草

11. *Bi Xie Shen Shi Tang* 萆薢渗湿汤
    Bi Xie (Rhizoma Dioscoreae Hypoglaucae) 萆薢
    Yi Ren (Semen Coicis) 薏仁
    Hua Shi (Talcum) 滑石
    Huang Bo (Cortex Phellodendri) 黄柏
    Fu Ling (Poria) 茯苓
    Dan Pi (Cortex Moutan) 丹皮
    Ze Xie (Rhizoma Alismatis) 泽泻
    Tong Cao (Medulla Tetrapanacis) 通草

12. *Bi Yan Pian* 鼻炎片
    Fang Feng (Radix Saposhnikoviae) 防风
    Jing Jie (Herba Schizpnepetac) 荆芥
    Cang Er Zi (Fructus Xanthii) 苍耳子
    Xin Yi (Flos Magnoliae) 辛夷
    Gan Cao (Radix Glycyrrhizae) 甘草
    Huang Bo (Cortex Phellodendri) 黄柏
    Xi Xin (Herba Asari) 细辛
    Ju Hua (Flos Chrisanthcmi) 菊花
    Zhi Mu (Rhizoma Anemarrhenae) 知母
    Jie Geng (Radix Platycodi) 桔梗
    Wu Wei Zi (Fructus Schisandrae) 五味子
    Ma Huang (Herba Ephedrae) 麻黄
    Lian Qiao (Fructus Forsythiae) 连翘
    Bai Zhi (Radix Angelicae Dahuricae) 白芷

13. *Brighten the Eyes**
    Dang Gui (Radix Angelicae Sinensis) 当归

Shu Di Huang (Radix Rehmanniae Praeparata) 熟地黄
Chuan Xiong (Rhizoma Chuanxiong) 川芎
Bai Shao (Radix Paeoniae Albae) 白芍
Qi Zi (Fructus Lycii) 杞子
Tu Si Zi (Semen Cuscutae) 菟丝子
Nu Zhen Zi (Fructus Ligustri Lucidi) 女贞子
Ju Hua (Flos Chrisanthemi) 菊花
Man Jing Zi (Fructus Viticis) 蔓荆子
Mi Meng Hua (Flos Buddleiae) 密蒙花
Ji Li (Fructus Tribuli) 蒺藜
Shou Wu (Radix Polygoni Multiflori) 首乌
Hong Zao (Fructus Jujubae) 红枣

14. *Brocade Sinews**
    Dang Shen (Radix Codonopsis) 党参
    Dang Gui (Radix Angelicae Sinensis) 当归
    Chuan Xiong (Rhizoma Chuanxiong) 川芎
    Bai Shao (Radix Paeoniae Albae) 白芍
    Shu Di Huang (Radix Rehmanniae Praeparata) 熟地黄
    Qi Zi (Fructus Lycii) 杞子
    Sang Ji Sheng (Herba Taxilli) 桑寄生
    Sang Zhi (Ramulis Mori) 桑枝
    Wei Ling Xian (Radix Clematidis) 威灵仙
    Mu Gua (Fructus Chaenomeus) 木瓜
    Wu Jia Pi (Cortex Acanthopanacis) 五加皮
    Xi Xian Cao (Herba Siegesbeckiae) 豨莶草
    Ji Xue Teng (Caulis Spatholobi) 鸡血藤
    Fu Ling (Poria) 茯苓
    Yi Ren (Semen Coicis) 薏仁
    Cang Zhu (Rhizoma Atractylodis) 苍术
    Zhi Gan Cao (Radix Glycyrrhizae Prep.) 炙甘草

15. *Bu Zhong Yi Qi Tang* 补中益气汤
    Huang Qi (Herba Ephedrae) 黄芪
    Ren Shen (Radix Ginseng) 人参
    Bai Zhu (Rhizoma Atractylodis Macrocephalae) 白术
    Gan Cao (Radix Glycyrrhizae) 甘草
    Chen Pi (Pericarpium Citrireticulatae) 陈皮
    Sheng Ma (Rhizoma Cimicifugae) 升麻
    Chai Hu (Radix Bupleuri) 柴胡
    Dang Gui (Radix Angelicae Sinensis) 当归

16. *Chai Ge Jie Ji Tang* 柴葛解肌汤
    Chai Hu (Radix Bupleuri) 柴胡
    Ge Gen (Radix Puerariae) 葛根

Shi Cao (Gypsum Fibrosum) 石膏

Huang Qin (Radix Scutellariae) 黄芩

Bai Shao (Radix Paeoniae Albae) 白芍

Qiang Huo (Rhizoma Seu Radix Notopterygii) 羌活

Bai Zhi (Radix Angelicae Dahuricae) 白芷

Gan Cao (Radix Glycyrrhizae) 甘草

Jie Geng (Radix Platycodi) 桔梗

Sheng Jiang (Rhizoma Zingiberis Recens) 生姜

Da Zao (Fructus Jujubae) 大枣

17. *Chai Hu Shu Gan Tang* 柴胡疏肝汤

Chai Hu (Radix Bupleuri) 柴胡

Bai Shao (Radix Paeoniae Albae) 白芍

Gan Cao (Radix Glycyrrhizae) 甘草

Zhi Qiao (Fructus Aurantii) 枳壳

Chen Pi (Pericarpium Citrireticulatae) 陈皮

Xiang Fu (Rhizoma Cyperi) 香附

Chuan Xiong (Rhizoma Chuanxiong) 川芎

18. *Chemo Support**

Huang Qi (Radix Astragali) 黄芪

Dang Shen (Radix Codonopsis Pilosulae) 党参

Tai Zi Shen (Radix Pseudostellariae) 太子参

Ling Zhi (Fructificatia Ganodermae Lucidi) 灵芝

Shan Yao (Rhizoma Dioscoreae) 山药

Xi Yang Shen (Radix Panacis Quinquefolii) 西洋参

Dan Pi (Cortex Moutan) 丹皮

Fu Ling (Poria) 茯苓

Chen Pi (Pericarpium Citri Reticulatae) 陈皮

Mai Dong (Radix Ophiopogonis) 麦冬

Dang Gui (Radix Angelicae Sinensis) 当归

Ban Xia (Rhizoma Pinelliae) 半夏

Lu Gen (Rhizoma Phragmitis) 芦根

Nu Zhen Zi (Fructus Ligustri Lucidi) 女贞子

Huang Jing (Rhizoma Polygonati) 黄精

Gan Cao (Radix Glycyrrhizae) 甘草

19. *Chi Feng Zhen Zhu An Chuang Wan* 彩凤珍珠暗疮丸

Zhen Zhu (Margarita) 珍珠

Zhen Zhu Mu (Concha Margaritifera Usta) 珍珠母

Shu Di Huang (Radix Rehmanniae) 熟地黄

Sha Shen (Radix Adenophorae Strictae) 沙参

Xuan Shen (Radix Scrophularriae) 玄参

Jin Yin Hua (Flos Lonicerae) 金银花

Huang Bo (Cortex Phellodendri) 黄柏

Da Huang (Radix Et Rhizoma Rhei) 大黄

20. *Chuan Bei Pi Pa Gao* 川贝枇杷膏
    Chuan Bei Mu (Bulbus Fritilariae Cirrhosae) 川贝母
    Pi Pa Ye (Folium Eriobotryae) 枇杷叶
    Sha Shen (Radix Adenophorae Strictae) 沙参
    Fu Ling (Poria) 茯苓
    Chen Pi (Pericarpium Citrireticulatae) 陈皮
    Jie Geng (Radix Platycodi) 桔梗
    Ban Xia (Rhizoma Pinelliae) 半夏
    Wu Wei Zi (Fructus Schisandrae) 五味子
    Gua Lou Ziu (Semen Trichosanthis) 瓜蒌仁
    Kuan Dong Hua (Flos Farfarae) 款冬花
    Yuan Zhi (Radix Polygalae) 远志
    Ku Xing Ren (Semen Armeniacae Amarum) 苦杏仁
    Sheng Jiang (Rhizoma Zingiberis Recens) 生姜
    Gan Cao (Radix Glycyrrhizae) 甘草
    Bo He (Herba Menthae) 薄荷

21. *Chuan Xiong Cha Tiao San* 川芎茶调散
    Bo He (Herba Menthae) 薄荷
    Xiang Fu (Rhizoma Cyperi) 香附
    Chuan Xiong (Rhizoma Chuanxiong) 川芎
    Jing Jie (Herba Schizpnepetae) 荆芥
    Fang Feng (Radix Saposhnikoviae) 防风
    Bai Zhi (Radix Angelicae Dahuricae) 白芷
    Qiang Huo (Rhizoma Seu Radix Notopterygii) 羌活
    Gan Cao (Radix Glycyrrhizae) 甘草

22. *Clear Lustre**
    Shou Wu (Radix Polygoni Multiflori) 首乌
    Dang Gui (Radix Angelicae Sinensis) 当归
    Bai Xian Pi (Cortex Dictamni) 白藓皮
    Fang Feng (Radix Ledebouriellae) 防风
    Jing Jie (Herba Schizonepetae) 荆芥
    Ju Hua (Flos Chrisanthemi) 菊花
    Ku Shen (Radix Sophorae Flavescentis) 苦参
    Dan Pi (Cortex Moutan) 丹皮
    Huang Qin (Radix Scutellariae) 黄芩
    Shi Gao (Gypsum Fibrosum) 石膏
    Zhi Mu (Rhizoma Anemarrhenae) 知母
    Gan Cao (Radix Glycyrrhizae) 甘草

23. *Clear the Soul*
    Zhu Ru (Caulis Bambusae in Taeniam) 竹茹
    Zhi Shi (Fructus Aurantii Immaturus) 枳实
    Ban Xia (Rhizoma Pinelliae) 半夏

Fu Ling (Poria) 茯苓
Chen Pi (Pericarpium Citri Reticulatae) 陈皮
Da Zao (Fructus Jujubae) 大枣
Gan Cao (Radix Glycyrrhizae) 甘草
He Huan Pi (Cortex Albizziae) 合欢皮
Yu Jin (Radix Curcumae) 郁金
Yuan Zhi (Radix Polygalae) 远志
Shi Chang Pu (Rhizoma Acori Tatarinowii) 石昌蒲
Bai Zi Ren (Semen Biotae) 柏子仁
Dan Shen (Radix Salviae Miltiorrhizae) 丹参

24. *Da Bu Yuan Jian* 大补元煎
Shu Di Huang (Radix Rehmanniae Prae.) 熟地黄
Shan Zhu Yu (Fructus Corni) 山茱萸
Shan Yao (Rhizoma Dioscoreae) 山药
Du Zhong (Cortex Eucommiae) 杜仲
Dang Gui (Radix Angelica Sinensis) 当归
Dang Shen (Radix Codonopsis Pilsulae) 党参
Qi Zi (Fructus Lycii) 杞子

25. *Da Chai Hu Tang* 大柴胡汤
Chai Hu (Radix Bupleuri) 柴胡
Huang Qin (Radix Scutellariae) 黄芩
Bai Shao (Radix Paeoniae Alba) 白芍
Ban Xia (Rhizoma Pinelliae) 半夏
Zhi Shi (Fructus Aurantii Immaturus) 枳实
Da Huang (Radix Et Rhizoma Rhei) 大黄
Sheng Jiang (Rhizoma Zingiberis Recens) 生姜
Da Zao (Fructus Jujubae) 大枣

26. *Da Cheng Qi Tang* 大承气汤
Da Huang (Radix Et Rhizoma Rhei) 大黄
Hou Po (Cortex Magnoliae Officinalis) 厚朴
Zhi Shi (Fructus Aurantii Immaturus) 枳实
Mang Xiao (Natrii Sulfas) 芒硝

27. *Da Qing Long Tang* 大青龙汤
Ma Huang (Herba Ephedrae) 麻黄
Ku Xing Ren (Semen Areniacae Amarum) 苦杏仁
Gan Cao (Radix Glycyrrhizae) 甘草
Gui Zhi (Ramulus Cinnamomi) 桂枝
Sheng Jiang (Rhizoma Zingiberis Recens) 生姜
Da Zao (Fructus Jujubae) 大枣
Shi Gao (Gypsum Fibrosum) 石膏

28. *Dan Shen Pian*   丹参片
    Dan Shen (Radix Salviae Miltiorrhizae)   丹参
    San Qi (Radix Notoginseng)   三七

29. *Dang Gui Si Ni Tang*   当归四逆汤
    Dang Gui (Radix Angelica Sinensis)   当归
    Gui Zhi (Ramulus Cinnamomi)   桂枝
    Bai Shao (Radix Pheoniae Alba)   白芍
    Xi Xin (Herba Asari)   细辛
    Gan Cao (Radix Glycyrrhizae)   甘草
    Mu Tong (Caulis Clematidis)   木通
    Da Zao (Fructus Jujubae)   大枣

30. *Dao Chi San*   导赤散
    Sheng Di Huang (Radix Rehmanniae)   生地黄
    Gan Cao (Radix Glycyrrhizae)   甘草
    Dan Zhu Ye (Herba Lophatheri)   淡竹叶
    Mu Tong (Caulis Clematidis)   木通

31. *Du Huo Ji Sheng Tang*   独活寄生汤
    Du Huo (Radix Angelicae Pubescens)   独活
    Sang Ji Sheng (Herba Taxilli)   桑寄生
    Du Zhong (Cortex Eucommiae)   杜仲
    Niu Xi (Radix Achyranthis Bidentatae)   牛膝
    Xi Xin (Herba Asari)   细辛
    Qin Jiao (Radix Gentianae Macrophyllae)   秦艽
    Fu Ling (Poria)   茯苓
    Fang Feng (Radix Saposhnikoviae)   防风
    Rou Gui (Cortex Cinnamomi)   肉桂
    Chuan Xiong (Rhizoma Chuanxiong)   川芎
    Ren Shen (Radix Ginseng)   人参
    Gan Cao (Radix Glycyrrhizae)   甘草
    Dang Gui (Radix Angelica Sinensis)   当归
    Bai Shao (Radix Pheoniae Alba)   白芍
    Shu Di Huang (Radix Rehmanniae Prae)   熟地黄

32. *Er Chen Tang*   二陈汤
    Ban Xia (Rhizoma Pinelliae)   半夏
    Chen Pi (Pericarpium Citri Reticulatae)   陈皮
    Fu Ling (Poria)   茯苓
    Gan Cao (Radix Glycyrrhizae)   甘草

33. *Er Ming Zuo Ci Wan*   耳鸣左慈丸
    Ci Shi (Magnetitum)   磁石
    Shan Zhu Yu (Fructus Corni)   山茱萸

Ze Xie (Rhizoma Alismatis)   泽泻
Dan Pi (Cortex Moutan)   丹皮
Sheng Di Huang (Radix Rehmanniae)   生地黄
Chai Hu (Radix Bupleuri)   柴胡
Wu Wei Zi (Fructus Schisandrae)   五味子
Shan Yao (Rhizoma Dioscoreae)   山药
Shu Di Huang (Radix Rehmanniae Prae.)   熟地黄
Ju Hua (Flos Chrisanthemi)   菊花
Tong Cao (Medulla Tetrapanacis)   通草

34. *Fang Feng Tong Sheng San*   防风通圣散
Fang Feng (Radix Saposhnikoviae)   防风
Jing Jie (Herba Schizonepetae)   荆芥
Bo He (Herba Menthae)   薄荷
Ma Huang (Herba Ephedrae)   麻黄
Da Huang (Radix Et Rhizoma Rhei)   大黄
Mang Xiao (Natrii Sulfas)   芒硝
Zhi Zi (Fructus Gardeniac)   栀子
Hua Shi (Talcum)   滑石
Jie Geng (Radix Platycodi)   桔梗
Shi Gao (Gypsum Fibrosum)   石膏
Chuan Xiong (Rhizoma Chuanxiong)   川芎
Dang Gui (Radix Angelica Sinensis)   当归
Bai Shao (Radix Paeomiae Alba)   白芍
Huang Qin (Radix Scutellariae)   黄芩
Lian Qiao (Fructus Forsythiae)   连翘
Bai Zhu (Rhizoma Atractylodis Macrocephalae)   白术
Gan Cao (Radix Glycyrrhizae)   甘草

35. *Freeing the Moon**
Chai Hu (Radix Bupleuri)   柴胡
Bo He (Herba Menthae)   薄荷
Dang Gui (Radix Angelicae Sinensis)   当归
Bai Shao (Radix Paeoniae Albae)   白芍
Dang Shen (Radix Codonopsis Pilosulae)   党参
Fu Ling (Poria)   茯苓
Qi Zi (Fructus Lycii)   杞子
Shou Wu (Radix Polygoni Multiflori)   首乌
Qin Pi (Pericarpium Citri Reticulatae Viride)   秦皮
He Huan Pi (Cortex Albizziae Sinensis)   合欢皮
Yuan Zhi (Radix Polygalae)   远志
Bai He (Bublus Lilii)   百合
Gan Cao (Radix Glycyrrhizae)   甘草
Hong Zao (Fructus Jujubae)   红枣
Ju Hua (Flos Chrisanthemi)   菊花

36. *Gan Mao Ling* 感冒灵
   Qing Hao (Herba Artemisia Annuae) 青蒿
   Qiang Huo (Rhizoma Seu Radix Notopterygii) 羌活
   Ban Lan Gen (Radix Isatidis) 板蓝根
   Ge Gen (Radix Puerariae) 葛根
   Mao Dong Qing (Radix Llicis Pubescentis) 毛冬青
   Ma Bian Cao (Herba Verbenae) 马鞭草
   Shi Gao (Gypsum Fibrosum) 石膏

37. *Ge Xia Zhu Yu Tang* 膈下逐瘀汤
   Dang Gui (Radix Angelicae Sinensis) 当归
   Chi Shao (Radix Paeonia Rubra) 赤芍
   Tao Ren (Semen Persicae) 桃仁
   Hong Hua (Flos Carthami) 红花
   Niun Xi (Radix Achyranthis Bidentatae) 牛膝
   Chai Hu (Radix Bupleuri) 柴胡
   Jie Geng (Radix Platycodi) 桔梗
   Zhi Qiao (Fructus Aurantii) 枳壳
   Sheng Di Huang (Radix Rehmanniae) 生地黄
   Gan Cao (Radix Glycyrrhizae) 甘草
   Chuen Xiong (Rhizoma Ligustici Chuanxiong) 川芎

38. *Glorious Sea** 当归
   Dang Gui (Radix Angelicae Sinensis) 当归
   Shou Wu (Radix Polygoni Multiflori) 首乌
   Qi Zi (Fructus Lycii) 杞子
   Bai Xian Pi (Cortex Dictami) 白藓皮
   Dan Pi (Cortex Moutan) 丹皮
   Huang Qin (Radix Scutellariae) 黄芩
   Tu Si Zi (Semen Cuscutae) 菟丝子
   Sheng Di Huang (Radix Rehmanniae) 生地黄
   Ze Xie (Rhizoma Alismatis) 泽泻
   Ban Xia (Rhizoma Pinelliae) 半夏
   Fu Ling (Poria) 茯苓
   Gan Cao (Radix Glycyrrhizae) 甘草

39. *Gui Pi Wan* 归脾丸
   Huang Qi (Radix Astragali) 黄芪
   Dang Shen (Radix Codonopsis Pilosulae) 党参
   Dang Gui (Radix Angelica Sinensis) 当归
   Long Yan Rou (Arillus Longan) 龙眼肉
   Bai Zhu (Rhizoma Atractylodis Macrocephalae) 白术
   Fu Ling (Poria) 茯苓
   Suan Zao Ren (Semen Ziziphi Spinosae) 酸枣仁
   Mu Xiang (Radix Acuklandiae) 木香

Yuan Zhi (Radix Polygalae)　　远志
Gan Cao (Radix Glycyrrhizae)　　甘草
Da Zao (Fructus Jujubae)　　大枣
Sheng Jiang (Rhizoma Zingiberis Recens)　　生姜

40.　*Gui Zhi Tang*　　桂枝汤
　　Gui Zhi (Ramulus Cinnamomi)　　桂枝
　　Bai Shao (Radix Paeoniae Alba)　　白芍
　　Gan Cao (Radix Glycyrrhizae)　　甘草
　　Sheng Jiang (Rhizoma Zingiberis Recens)　　生姜
　　Da Zao (Fructus Jujubae)　　大枣

41.　*Huang Qi Jian Zhong Tang*　　黄芪建中汤
　　Gui Zhi (Ramulus Cinnamomi)　　桂枝
　　Bai Shao (Radix Paeoniae Alba)　　白芍
　　Gan Cao (Radix Glycyrrhizae)　　甘草
　　Sheng Jiang (Rhizoma Zingiberis Recens)　　生姜
　　Da Zao (Fructus Jujubae)　　大枣
　　Huang Qi (Radix Astragali)　　黄芪
　　Yi Tang (Saccharum Granorum)　　饴糖

42.　*Huo Xiang Zheng Qi Wan*　　藿香正气丸
　　Huo Xiang (Herba Agastachis)　　藿香
　　Ban Xia (Rhizoma Pinelliae)　　半夏
　　Hou Po (Cortex Magnoliae Officinalis)　　厚朴
　　Su Ye (Folium Perillae)　　苏叶
　　Bai Zhi (Radix Angelicae Dahuricae)　　白芷
　　Da Fu Pi (Pericarpium Arecae)　　大腹皮
　　Jie Geng (Radix Platycodi)　　桔梗
　　Gan Cao (Radix Glycyrrhizae)　　甘草

43.　*Jade Spring**　
　　Bei Sha Shen (Radix Glehniae)　　北沙参
　　Mai Dong (Radix Ophiopogonis)　　麦冬
　　Yu Zhu (Rhizoma Polygonati Odorati)　　玉竹
　　Gan Cao (Radix Glycyrrhizae)　　甘草
　　Sang Ye (Folium Mori)　　桑叶
　　Bian Dou (Semen Lablab Album)　　扁豆
　　Tian Hua Fen (Radix Trichosanthis)　　天花粉
　　Shi Hu (Herba Dendrobii)　　石斛
　　Tai Zi Shen (Radix Pseudostellariae)　　太子参
　　Dang Shen (Radix Codonopsis)　　丹参
　　Fu Ling (Poria)　　茯苓
　　Zhi Mu (Rhizoma Anemarrhenae)　　知母
　　Shan Yao (Rhizoma Dioscoreae)　　山药

44. *Jin Suo Gu Jing Wan*   金锁固精丸
     Ji Li (Fructus Tribuli)   蒺藜
     Qian Shi (Semen Euryalis)   芡实
     Lian Zi (Semen Nelumbinis)   莲子
     Lian Xu (Stamen Nelumbinis)   莲须
     Long Gu (Os Draconis)   龙骨
     Mu Li (Concha Ostreae)   牡蛎

45. *Jing Fang Bai Du San*   荆防败毒散
     Fang Feng (Radix Saposhnikoviae)   防风
     Jing Jie (Herba Schizonepetae)   荆芥
     Tu Fu Ling (Rhizoma Smilacis Glabrae)   土茯苓
     Qiang Huo (Rhizoma Seu Radix Notopterygii)   羌活
     Du Huo (Radix Angelicae Pubescens)   独活
     Chuan Xiong (Rhizoma Chuanxiong)   川芎
     Chai Hu (Radix Bupleuri)   柴胡
     Bo He (Herba Menthae)   薄荷
     Qian Hu (Radix Peucedani)   前胡
     Jie Geng (Radix Platycodi)   桔梗
     Zhi Qiao (Fructus Aurantii)   枳壳
     Dang Shen (Radix Codonopsis Piolosulae)   党参
     Gan Cao (Radix Glycyrrhizae)   甘草

46. *Jiu Wei Qiang Huo Wan*   九味羌活丸
     Qiang Huo (Rhizoma Seu Radix Notopterygii)   羌活
     Fang Feng (Radix Saposhnikoviae)   防风
     Cang Zhu (Rhizoma Atractylodis)   苍术
     Xi Xin (Herba Asari)   细辛
     Chuan Xiong (Rhizoma Chuanxiong)   川芎
     Bai Zhi (Radix Angelicae Dahuricae)   白芷
     Huang Qin (Radix Scutellariae)   黄芩
     Di Huang (Radix Rehmanniae)   地黄
     Gan Cao (Radix Glycyrrhizae)   甘草

47. *Li Zhong Wan*   理中丸
     Gan Jing (Rhizoma Zingiberis)   干姜
     Bai Zhu (Rhizoma Atractylodis Macrocephalae)   白术
     Dang Shen (Radix Codonopsis Pilosulae)   党参
     Gan Cao (Radix Glycyrrhizae)   甘草

48. *Liu Wei Di Huang Wan*   六味地黄丸
     Shu Di Huang (Radix Rehmanniae Prae.)   熟地黄
     Shan Yao (Rhizoma Dioscoreae)   山药
     Ze Xie (Rhizoma Alismatis)   泽泻
     Dan Pi (Cortex Moutan)   丹皮

Fu Ling (Poria)　　　　　　　　　　　　　　　　　茯苓
Zhi Mu (Rhizoma Anemarrhenae)　　　　　　　　　知母
Huang Bo (Cortex Phellodendri)　　　　　　　　　黄柏

49.　*Liu Yi San*　　　　　　　　　　　　　　　　　六一散
Hua Shi (Talcum)　　　　　　　　　　　　　　　　滑石
Gan Cao (Radix Glycyrrhizae)　　　　　　　　　　甘草

50.　*Long Dan Xie Gan Tang*　　　　　　　　　　　龙胆泻肝汤
Long Dan Cao (Radix Gentiana)　　　　　　　　　龙胆草
Huang Qin (Radix Scutellariae)　　　　　　　　　黄芩
Zhi Zi (Fructus Gardeniae)　　　　　　　　　　　栀子
Ze Xie (Rhizoma Alismatis)　　　　　　　　　　　泽泻
Mu Tong (Caulis Clematidis)　　　　　　　　　　木通
Che Qian Zi (Semen Plantaginis)　　　　　　　　车前子
Dang Gui (Radix Angelica Sinensis)　　　　　　　当归
Sheng Di Huang (Radix Rehmanniae)　　　　　　　生地黄
Chai Hu (Radix Bupleuri)　　　　　　　　　　　　柴胡
Gan Cao (Radix Glycyrrhizae)　　　　　　　　　　甘草

51.　*Ma Huang Tang*　　　　　　　　　　　　　　麻黄汤
Ma Huang (Herba Ephedrae)　　　　　　　　　　　麻黄
Gui Zhi (Ramulus Cinnamomi)　　　　　　　　　　桂枝
Ku Xing Ren (Semen Armeniacae Amarum)　　　　苦杏仁
Gan Cao (Radix Glycyrrhizae)　　　　　　　　　　甘草

52.　*Ma Xing Shi Gan Tang*　　　　　　　　　　　麻杏石甘汤
Ma Huang (Herba Ephedrae)　　　　　　　　　　　麻黄
Ku Xing Ren (Semen Armeniacae Amarum)　　　　苦杏仁
Gan Cao (Radix Glycyrrhizae)　　　　　　　　　　甘草
Shi Gao (Gypsum Fibrosum)　　　　　　　　　　　石膏

53.　*Ma Xing Yi Gan Tang*　　　　　　　　　　　麻杏薏甘汤
Ma Huang (Herba Ephedrae)　　　　　　　　　　　麻黄
Ku Xing Ren (Semen Armeniacae Amarum)　　　　苦杏仁
Gan Cao (Radix Glycyrrhizae)　　　　　　　　　　甘草
Yi Ren (Semen Coicis)　　　　　　　　　　　　　薏仁

54.　*Ma Zi Ren Tang*　　　　　　　　　　　　　　麻子仁汤
Ma Huang (Herba Ephedrae)　　　　　　　　　　　麻黄
Bai Shao (Radix Paeoniae Alba)　　　　　　　　　白芍
Zhi Shi (Fructus Aurantii Immaturus)　　　　　　枳实
Da Huang (Radix Et Rhizoma Rhei)　　　　　　　大黄
Hou Po (Cortex Magnoliae Officinalis)　　　　　厚朴
Ku Xing Ren (Semen Armeniacae Ararum)　　　　苦杏仁

55. *Ming Mu Di Huang Wan* 明目地黄丸
    Shu Di Huang (Radix Rehmanniae Prae.) 熟地黄
    Shan Zhu Yu (Fructus Corni) 山茱萸
    Qi Zi (Fructus Lycii) 杞子
    Shan Yao (Rhizoma Dioscoreae) 山药
    Dang Gui (Radix Angelica Sinensis) 当归
    Bai Shao (Radix Paeoniae Alba) 白芍
    Dan Pi (Cortex Moutan) 丹皮
    Ji Li (Fructus Tribuli) 蒺藜
    Shi Jue Ming (Concha Haliotidis) 石决明
    Fu Ling (Poria) 茯苓
    Ze Xie (Rhizoma Alismatis) 泽泻
    Ju Hua (Flos Chrisanthemi) 菊花

56. *Open the Heart**
    Ban Xia (Rhizoma Pinelliae) 半夏
    Hou Po (Cortex Magnoliae Officinalis) 厚朴
    Zi Su Ye (Folium Perillae) 紫苏叶
    Da Zao (Fructus Jujubae) 大枣
    Gan Cao (Radix Glycyrrhizae) 甘草
    Chai Hu (Radix Bupleuri) 柴胡
    Bai He (Bulbus Lilli) 百合
    Jie Geng (Radix Platycodi) 桔梗
    Qing Pi (Pericarpium Citri Reticulatae Viride) 青皮
    He Huan Pi (Cortex Albizziae) 合欢皮

57. *Ping Wei San* 平胃散
    Chen Pi (Pericarpium Citri Reticulatae) 陈皮
    Hou Po (Cortex Magnoliae Officinalis) 厚朴
    Cang Zhu (Rhizoma Atractylodis) 苍术
    Gan Cao (Radix Glycyrrhzae) 甘草
    Sheng Jiang (Rhizoma Zingiberis Recens) 生姜
    Da Zao (Fructus Jujubae) 大枣

58. *Qi Ju Di Huang Wan* 杞菊地黄丸
    Shu Di Huang (Radix Rehmanniae Prae.) 熟地黄
    Qi Zi (Fructus Lycii) 杞子
    Shan Yao (Rhizoma Dioscoreae) 山药
    Shan Zhu Yu (Fructus Corni) 山茱萸
    Fu Ling (Poria) 茯苓
    Dan Pi (Cortex Moutan) 丹皮
    Ze Xie (Rhizoma Alismatis) 泽泻
    Ju Hua (Flos Chrisanthemi) 菊花

59. *Qing Qi Hua Tan Wan* 清气化痰丸
Da Huang (Radix Et Rhizoma Rhei) 大黄
Huang Qin (Radix Scutellariae) 黄芩
Huang Lian (Rhizoma Coptidis) 黄连
Xuan Shen (Radix Scrophulariae) 玄参
Qing Dai (Indico Naturalis) 青黛
Xiang Fu (Rhizoma Cyperi) 香附
Zhi Shi (Fructus Aurantii Immaturus) 枳实
Shan Zha (Fructus Crataegi) 山楂
Gua Lou Zi (Semen Trichosanthis) 瓜蒌子
Su Zi (Fructus Perillae) 苏子
Lai Fu Zi (Semen Raphani) 莱服子
Chen Pi (Pericarpium Citri Reticulatae) 陈皮
Ban Xia (Rhizoma Pinelliae) 半夏
Fu Ling (Poria) 茯苓
Bai Zhu (Rhizoma Atractylodis Macrocephalae) 白术
Zhe Bei Mu (Bulbus Fritillariae Thunbergii) 浙贝母
Fu Hai Shi (Pumex) 浮海石
Bai Bu (Radix Stemonae) 百部
Tian Nan Xing (Rhizoma Asisaematis) 天南星

60. *Qing Wei San* 清胃散
Dang Gui (Radix Angelica Sinensis) 当归
Sheng Ma (Rhizoma Cimicifugae) 升麻
Huang Lian (Rhizoma Coptidis) 黄连
Sheng Di Huang (Radix Rehmanniae) 生地黄
Dan Pi (Cortex Moutan) 丹皮

61. *Radio Support**
Huang Qi (Radix Astragali) 黄芪
Dang Gui (Radix Angelicae Sinensis) 当归
Hong Hua (Flos Carthami) 红花
Dan Shen (Radix Salviae Miltiorrhizae) 丹参
Tai Zi Shen (Radix Pseudostellariae) 太子参
Shou Wu (Radix Polygoni Multiflori) 首乌
Qi Zi (Fructus Lycii) 杞子
Wu Wei Zi (Fructus Schisandrae) 五味子
Nu Zhen Zi (Fructus Ligustri Lucidi) 女贞子
Zhi Mu (Rhizoma Anemarrhenae) 知母
Dan Pi (Cortex Moutan) 丹皮
Chi Shao (Radix Paeoniae Rubrae) 赤芍
Gan Cao (Radix Glycyrrhizae) 甘草

62. *Red Stirring**

    Dang Gui (Radix Angelicae Sinensis) 当归
    Sheng Di Huang (Radix Rehmanniae) 生地黄
    Chuan Xiong (Rhizoma Chuanxiong) 川芎
    Chi Shao (Radix Paeoniae Rubrae) 赤芍
    Tao Ren (Semen Persicae) 桃仁
    Hong Hua (Flos Carthami) 红花
    Chai Hu (Radix Bupleuri) 柴胡
    Zhi Qiao (Fructus Aurantii) 枳壳
    Niu Xi (Radix Achyranthis Bidentatae) 牛膝
    Jie Geng (Radix Platycodi) 桔梗
    Gan Cao (Radix Glycyrrhizae) 甘草
    Dan Shen (Radix Salviae Miltiorrhizae) 丹参
    Yuan Zhi (Radix Polygalae) 远志
    Yu Jin (Radix Curcumae) 郁金
    He Huan Pi (Cortex Albizziae) 合欢皮

63. *Release Constraint**

    Xiang Fu (Rhizoma Cyperi) 香附
    Chuan Xiong (Rhizoma Chuanxiong) 川芎
    Cang Zhu (Rhizoma Atractylodis) 苍术
    Zhi Zi (Fructus Gardeniae) 栀子
    Shen Qu (Massa Fermantata Medicinalis) 神曲
    He Huan Pi (Cortex Albizziae) 合欢皮
    Shi Chang Pu (Rhizoma Acori Tatarinowii) 石菖蒲
    Gan Cao (Radix Glycyrrhizae) 甘草

64. *Ren Shen Yang Rong Wan* 人参养荣丸

    Ren Shen (Radix Ginseng) 人参
    Bai Zhu (Rhizoma Atractylodis Macrocephalae) 白术
    Fu Ling (Poria) 茯苓
    Gan Cao (Radix Glycyrrhizae) 甘草
    Huang Qi (Radix Astragali) 黄芪
    Shu Di Huang (Radix Rehmanniae Prae.) 熟地黄
    Dang Gui (Radix Angelica Sinensis) 当归
    Bai Shao (Radix Paeoniae Alba) 白芍
    Rou Gui (Cortex Cinnamomi) 肉桂
    Chen Pi (Pericarpium Citri Reticulatae) 陈皮
    Yuan Zhi (Radix Polygalae) 远志
    Wu Wei Zi (Fructus Schisandrae) 五味子

65. *Root the Spirit**

    Bai Shao (Radix Paeoniae Albae) 白芍
    Dang Gui (Radix Angelicae Sinensis) 当归
    Long Gu (Os Draconis) 龙骨
    Tu Si Zi (Semen Cuscutae) 菟丝子

Mai Dong (Radix Ophiopogonis) 麦冬
Bai Zi Ren (Semen Biotae) 柏子仁
Suan Zao Ren (Semen Ziziphi Spinosae) 酸枣仁
Fu Ling (Poria) 茯苓

66. *Run Chang Wan* 润肠丸
Da Huang (Radix Et Rhizoma Rhei) 大黄
Qiang Huo (Rhizoma Seu Radix Notopterygii) 羌活
Ma Ren (Fructus Cannabis) 麻仁
Dang Gui (Radix Angellica Sinensis) 当归
Tao Ren (Semen Persicae) 桃仁

67. *San Huang Shi Gao Tang* 三黄石膏汤
Da Huang (Radix Et Rhizoma Rhei) 大黄
Huang Lian (Rhizoma Coptidis) 黄连
Huang Qin (Radix Scutellariae) 黄芩
Shi Gao (Gypsum Fibrosum) 石膏

68. *Sang Ju Gan Mao Pian* 桑菊感冒丸
Sang Ye (Folium Mori) 桑叶
Ju Hua (Flos Christanthemi) 菊花
Bo He (Herba Menthae) 薄荷
Ku Xing Ren (Semen Armeniacae Amarum) 苦杏仁
Jie Geng (Radix Platycodi) 桔梗
Lian Qiao (Fructus Forsythiae) 连翘
Lu Gen (Rhizoma Phragmitis) 芦根
Gan Cao (Radix Glycyrrihizae) 甘草

69. *Sang Ju Yin* 桑菊饮
Sang Ye (Folium Mori) 桑叶
Ju Hua (Flos Chrisanthemi) 菊花
Lian Qiao (Fructus Forsythiae) 连翘
Ku Xing Ren (Semen Armeniacac Amarum) 苦杏仁
Lu Gan (Rhizoma Phragmitis) 芦根
Bo He (Herba Menthae) 薄荷
Jie Geng (Radix Platycodi) 桔梗
Gan Cao (Radix Glycyrrhizae) 甘草

70. *Sha Shen Mai Dong Tang* 沙参麦冬汤
Sha Shen (Radix Adenophorae Strictae) 沙参
Mai Dong (Radix Ophiopogonis) 麦冬
Yu Zhu (Rhizoma Polygonati Odorati) 玉竹
Gan Cao (Radix Glycyrrhizae) 甘草
Sang Ye (Folium Mori) 桑叶
Bian Dou (Semen Dolichoris) 扁豆
Tian Hua Fen (Radix Trichosanthis) 天花粉

71. *Sheng Mai San*   生脉散
    Ren Shen (Radix Ginseng)   人参
    Mai Dong (Radix Ophiopogonis)   麦冬
    Wu Wei Zi (Fructus Schisandrae)   五味子

72. *Shi Chuan Da Bu Wan*   十全大补丸
    Ren Shen (Radix Ginseng)   人参
    Bai Zhu (Rhizoma Atractylodis Macrocephalae)   白术
    Fu Ling (Poria)   茯苓
    Gan Cao (Radix Glycyrrhizae)   甘草
    Dang Gui (Radix Angelica Sinensis)   当归
    Shu Di Huang (Radix Rehmanniae Prae.)   熟地黄
    Bai Shao (Radix Paeoniae Alba)   白芍
    Chuan Xiong (Rhizoma Chuanxiong)   川芎
    Huang Qi (Radix Astragali)   黄芪
    Rou Gui (Cortex Cinnamomi)   肉桂

73. *Si Jun Zi Tang*   四君子汤
    Dang Shen (Radix Codonopsis Pilosulae)   党参
    Bai Zhu (Rhizoma Atractylodis Macrocephalae)   白术
    Fu Ling (Poria)   茯苓
    Gan Cao (Radix Glycyrrhizae)   甘草

74. *Si Miao Yong An Tang*   四妙勇安汤
    Jin Yin Hua (Flos Lonicerae)   金银花
    Xuan Shen (Radix Scrophulariae)   玄参
    Dang Gui (Radix Angelica Sinensis)   当归
    Gan Cao (Radix Glycyrrhizae)   甘草

75. *Si Ni San*   四逆散
    Chai Hu (Radix Bupleuri)   柴胡
    Zhi Shi (Fructus Aurantii Immaturus)   枳实
    Bai Shao (Radix Paeoniae Alba)   白芍
    Gan Cao (Radix Glycyrrhizae)   甘草

76. *Si Wu Tang*   四物汤
    Shu Di Huang (Radix Rehmanniae Prae.)   熟地黄
    Dang Gui (Radix Angelicae Sinensis)   当归
    Bai Shao (Radix Paeoniae Alba)   白芍
    Chuan Xiong (Rhizoma Chuanxiong)   川芎

77. *Stir Field of Elixir**
    Wu Yao (Radix Linderae)   乌药
    Dang Gui (Radix Angelicae Sinensis)   当归
    Chuan Xiong (Rhizoma Chuanxiong)   川芎

Tao Ren (Semen Persicae) 桃仁
Dan Pi (Cortex Moutan) 丹皮
Chi Shao (Radix Paeoniae Rubrae) 赤芍
Yuan Hu (Rhizoma Corydalis) 元胡
Gan Cao (Radix Glycyrrhizae) 甘草
Xiang Fu (Rhizoma Cyperi) 香附
Hong Hua (Flos Corthami) 红花
Zhi Qiao (Fructus Aurantii) 枳壳
Pu Huang (Pollen Typhae) 蒲黄
Dan Shen (Radix Salciae Miltiorrhizae) 丹参
Bai Shao (Radix Paeomiae Albae) 白芍

78. *Strengthen the Root**
Shu Di Huang (Radix Rehmanniae Prae.) 熟地黄
Shan Yao (Rhizoma Dioscoreae) 山药
Shan Zhu Yu (Fructus Corni) 山茱萸
Qi Zi (Fructus Lycii) 杞子
Lu Rong (Cornu Cervi Pantotrichum) 鹿茸
Tu Si Zi (Semen Cuscutae) 菟丝子
Du Zhong (Cortex Eucommiae) 杜仲
Dang Gui (Radix Angelicae Sinensis) 当归
Rou Gui (Cortex Cinnamomi) 肉桂
Gui Zhi (Ramulus Cinnamomi) 桂枝
Zhi Gan Cao (Radix Glycyrrhizae Prae.) 炙甘草
Ren Shen (Radix Ginseng) 人参
Zhi Mu (Rhizoma Anemarrheae) 知母

79. *Tong Bi Wan* 通鼻丸
Cang Er Zi (Fructus Xanthii) 苍耳子
Xin Yi (Flos Magnoliae) 辛夷
Lu Gen (Rhizoma Phragmitis) 芦根
Gan Cao (Radix Glycyrrhizae) 甘草
Jie Geng (Radix Platycodi) 桔梗
Sang Ye (Folium Mori) 桑叶

80. *Wen Dan Tang* 温胆汤
Zhu Ru (Caulis Bambusae in Taeniam) 竹茹
Zhi Shi (Fructus Aurantii Immaturus) 枳实
Ban Xia (Rhizoma Pinelliae) 半夏
Fu Ling (Poria) 茯苓
Chen Pi (Pericarpium Citri Reticulatae) 陈皮
Da Zao (Fructus Ziziphi Jujubae) 大枣
Gan Cao (Radix Glycyrrhizae) 甘草
Sheng Jiang (Rhizoma Zingiberis Recens) 生姜

81. *Wen Jing Tang* 温经汤
   Wu Zhu Yu (Fructus Evodiae) 吴茱萸
   Gui Zhi (Ramulus Cinnamomi) 桂枝
   Dang Gui (Radix Angelicae Sinensis) 当归
   Chuan Xiong (Rhizoma Chuanxiong) 川芎
   Bai Shao (Radix Paeoniae Alba) 白芍
   E Jiao (Colla Corii Asini) 阿胶
   Mai Dong (Radix Ophiopogonis) 麦冬
   Dan Pi (Cortex Moutan Radicis) 丹皮
   Ren Shen (Radix Ginseng) 人参
   Gan Cao (Radix Glycyrrhizae) 甘草
   Ban Xia (Rhizoma Pinelliae) 半夏
   Sheng Jiang (Rhizoma Zingiberis Recens) 生姜

82. *Wu Ji Bai Feng Wan* 乌鸡白凤丸
   Wu Ji (Black meat chicken) 乌鸡
   Dang Gui (Radix Angelicae Sinensis) 当归
   Bai Shao (Radix Paeoniae Alba) 白芍
   Sheng Di Huang (Radix Rehmanniae) 生地黄
   Shu Di Huang (Radix Rehmanniae Prae.) 熟地黄
   Chuan Xiong (Rhizoma Chuanxiong) 川芎
   Huang Qi (Radix Astragali) 黄芪
   Xiang Fu (Rhizoma Cyperi) 香附
   Dan Shen (Radix Salviae Miltiorrhizae) 丹参
   Mu Li (Concha Ostreae) 牡蛎
   Chai Hu (Radix Bupleuri) 柴胡
   Tian Dong (Radix Asparagi) 天冬
   Lu Jiao Shuang (Cornu Cervi Degelatinatum) 鹿角霜
   Lu Jiao Jiao (Colla Cornus Cervi) 鹿角胶
   Sang Piao Xiao (Ootheca Mantidis) 桑螵蛸
   Qian Shi (Semen Euryalis) 芡实
   Shan Yao (Rhizoma Dioscoreae) 山药
   Gan Cao (Radix Glycyrrhizae) 甘草
   Ren Shen (Radix Ginseng) 人参

83. *Wu Ling San* 五苓散
   Fu Ling (Poria) 茯苓
   Zhu Ling (Polyporus) 猪苓
   Bai Zhu (Rhizoma Atractylodis Macrocephalae) 白术
   Ze Xie (Rhizoma Alismatis) 泽泻
   Gui Zhi (Ramulus Cinnamomi) 桂枝

84. *Wu Mei Wan* 乌梅丸
   Wu Mei (Fructus Mume) 乌梅
   Huang Lian (Rhizoma Coptidis) 黄连

Huang Bo (Cortex Phellodendri) 黄柏
Gan Jiang (Rhizoma Zingiberis) 干姜
Shu Jiao (Pericarpium Znathoxyli) 蜀椒
Gui Zhi (Ramulus Cinnamomi) 桂枝
Fu Zi (Radix Aconiti Prae.) 附子
Dang Gui (Radix Angelicae Sinensis) 当归
Ren Shen (Radix Ginseng) 人参
Xi Xin (Herba Asari) 细辛

85. *Xiang Sha Liu Jun Zi Wan* 香砂六君子丸
Ren Shen (Radix Ginseng) 人参
Bai Zhu (Rhizoma Atractylodis Macrocephalae) 白术
Fu Ling (Poria) 茯苓
Chen Pi (Pericarpium Citri Reticutatae) 陈皮
Ban Xia (Rhizoma Pinelliae) 半夏
Mu Xiang (Radix Aucklandiae) 木香
Sha Ren (Fructus Amomi) 砂仁
Gan Cao (Radix Glycyrrhizae) 甘草

86. *Xiang Sha Yang Wei Tang* 香砂养胃汤
Bai Zhu (Rhizoma Atractylodis Macrocephalae) 白术
Xiang Fu (Rhizoma Cyeri) 香附
Chen Pi (Pericarpium Citri Reticutatae) 陈皮
Huo Xiang (Herba Agastachis) 藿香
Fu Ling (Poria) 茯苓
Dou Kou (Fructus Amomi Rotundus) 豆蔻
Hou Po (Cortex Magnoliac Officinalis) 厚朴
Zhi Shi (Fructus Aurantii Immaturus) 枳实
Ban Xia (Rhizoma Pinelliae) 半夏
Mu Xing (Radix Aucklandiae) 木香
Sha Ren (Fructus Amomi) 砂仁
Gan Cao (Radix Glycyrrhizae) 甘草

87. *Xiao Chai Hu Tang* 小柴胡汤
Chai Hu (Radix Bupleuri) 柴胡
Huang Qin (Radix Scutellariae) 黄芩
Sheng Jiang (Rhizoma Zingiberis Recens) 生姜
Ren Shen (Radix Ginseng) 人参
Da Zao (Fructus Jujubae) 大枣
Gan Cao (Radix Glycyrrhizae) 甘草

88. *Xiao Qing Long Tang* 小青龙汤
Ma Huang (Herba Ephedrae) 麻黄
Bai Shao (Radix Paeoniae Alba) 白芍
Gui Zhi (Ramulus Cinnamomi) 桂枝

Ban Xia (Rhizoma Pinelliae)   半夏
Gan Jiang (Rhizoma Zingiberis)   干姜
Wu Wei Zi (Fructus Schisandrae)   五味子
Xi Xin (Herba Asari)   细辛
Gan Cao (Radix Glycyrrhizae)   甘草

89. *Xiao Yao Wan*   逍遥丸
Chai Hu (Radix Bupleuri)   柴胡
Dang Gui (Radix Angelica Sinensis)   当归
Bai Zhu (Rhizoma Atractylodis Macrocephalae)   白术
Bai Shao (Radix Paeoniae Alba)   白芍
Fu Ling (Poria)   茯苓
Gan Cao (Radix Glycyrrhizae)   甘草
Sheng Jiang (Rhizoma Zingiberis Recens)   生姜
Bo He (Herba Menthae)   薄荷

90. *Xue Fu Zhu Yu Tang*   血府逐瘀汤
Dang Gui (Radix Angelica Sinensis)   当归
Sheng Di Huang (Radix Rehmanniae)   生地黄
Chuan Xiong (Rhizoma Chuanxiong)   川芎
Chi Shao (Radix Paeonia Rubra)   赤芍
Tao Ren (Semen Persicae)   桃仁
Hong Hua (Flos Carthami)   红花
Chai Hu (Radix Bupleuri)   柴胡
Zhi Qiao (Fructus Aurantii)   枳壳
Niu Xi (Radix Achyranthis Bidentatae)   牛膝
Jie Geng (Radix Platycodi)   桔梗
Gan Cao (Radix Glycyrrhizae)   甘草

91. *Yin Chen Tang*   茵陈汤
Yin Chen (Herba artemisiae Scopariae)   茵陈
Zhi Zi (Fructus Gardeniae)   栀子
Da Huang (Radix Et Rhizoma Rhei)   大黄

92. *Yin Chen Wu Ling San*   茵陈五苓散
Yin Chen (Herba Artemisiae Scopariae)   茵陈
Fu Ling (Poria)   茯苓
Zhu Ling (Polyporus)   猪苓
Bai Zhu (Rhizoma Atractylodis Macrocephalae)   白术
Ze Xie (Rhizoma Alismatis)   泽泻
Gui Zhi (Ramulus Cinnamomi)   桂枝

93. *Yin Qiao Jie Du Pian*   银翘解毒片
Jin Yin Hua (Flos Lonicerae)   金银花
Lian Qiao (Fructus Forysthiae)   连翘

Niu Bang Zi (Fructus Arctii) 牛蒡子
Dan Dou Chi (Semen Sojae Prae.) 淡豆豉
Dan Zhu Ye (Herba Lophatheri) 淡竹叶
Lu Gen (Rhizoma Phragmitis) 卢根
Jie Geng (Radix Platycodi) 桔梗
Bo He (Herba Menthae) 薄荷
Jing Jie (Herba Schizonepetae) 荆芥
Gan Cao (Radix Glycyrrhizae) 甘草

94. *You Gui Yin* 右归饮
Shu Di Huang (Radix Rehmanniae Prae.) 熟地黄
Shan Yao (Rhizoma Dioscoreae) 山药
Shan Zhu Yu (Fructus corni) 山茱萸
Du Zhong (Cortex Eucommiae) 杜仲
Qi Zi (Fructus Lycii) 杞子
Fu Zi (Radix Aconiti Prae.) 附子
Rou Gui (Cortex Cinnamomi) 肉桂
Gan Cao (Radix Glycyrrhizae) 甘草

95. *Yu Nu Jian* 玉女煎
Shi Gao (Gpysum Fibrosum) 石膏
Shu Di Huang (Radix Rehmanniae Prae.) 熟地黄
Mai Dong (Radix Ophiopogonis) 麦冬
Niu Xi (Radix Achyranthis Bidentatae) 牛膝
Zhi Mu (Rhizoma Anemarrhenae) 知母

96. *Yue Ju Wan* 越鞠丸
Xiang Fu (Rhizoma Cyperi) 香附
Chuan Xiong (Rhizoma Chuanxiong) 川芎
Cang Zhu (Rhizoma Atractylodis) 苍术
Zhi Zi (Fructus Gardeniae) 栀子
Shen Qu (Massa Fermantala Medicinalis) 神曲

97. *Zhen Zhu San* 珍珠散
Zhen Zhu (Margarita) 珍珠

98. *Zhi Bo Di Huang Wan* 知柏地黄丸
Zhi Mu (Rhizoma Anemarrhenae) 知母
Huang Bo (Cortex Phellodendri) 黄柏
Shu Di Huang (Radix Rehmanniae Prae.) 熟地黄
Shan Zhu Yu (Fructus Corni) 山茱萸
Dan Pi (Cortex Moutan) 丹皮
Shan Yao (Rhizoma Dioscoreae) 山药
Fu Ling (Poria) 茯苓
Ze Xie (Rhizoma Alismatis) 泽泻

99. *Zhu Ling Tang* 猪苓汤
   Zhu Ling (Polyporus) 猪苓
   Fu Ling (Poria) 茯苓
   Ze Xie (Rhizoma Alismatis) 泽泻
   E Jiao (Colla Corii Asini) 阿胶
   Hua Shi (Talcum) 滑石

100. *Zuo Gui Wan* 左归丸
   Shu Di Huang (Radix Rehmanniae Prae.) 熟地黄
   Shan Yao (Rhizoma Dioscoreae) 山药
   Qi Zi (Fructus Lycii) 杞子
   Tu Si Zi (Semen Cuscutae) 菟丝子
   Lu Jiao Jiao (Cervus Nippon) 鹿角胶
   Niu Xi (Radix Achyranthis Bidentatae) 牛膝

101. *Zuo Jin Wan* 左金丸
   Huang Lian (Rhizoma Coptidis) 黄连
   Wu Zhu Yu (Fructus Evodiae) 吴茱萸

*The formulae of these Chinese Ready-made Medicines are created in the handbook entitled "The Three Treasures" in which only the English names are given. (See Reference 24, Chapter 7).

INDEX FOR GENERAL PRINCIPLES

Index for List of Pin Yin Name of Chinese Medicinal Herbs

Index for List of Herbs According to Orthodox Indications

(2) Cardiotonic Herbs 强心药

D. Nervous System 神经系统

F.   Tonics Herbs 补益药

G.   Anti-inflammatory Herbs 抗炎症药

H. Antidiabetic Herbs 降血糖药

I.   Antibacterial Herbs 抗细菌药

J. Antiviral Herbs 抗病毒药

K. Antimycotic Herbs 抗真菌药

L. Antimalara Herbs 抗疟疾药

M. Antiamebial Herbs 抗阿米巴药

P. Photosensitizer Herbs 对光敏感药

Index for List of Latin Names of Chinese Medicinal Herbs

18. Anthelmitics 驱虫药